HOLISTIC EDUCATION:

Teaching of Science in the Affective Domain

by
ISADORE L. SONNIER

Philosophical Library
New York

Library of Congress Cataloging in Publication Data

Sonnier, Isadore L.
  Holistic education.

  Bibliography: p.
  1. Science—Study and teaching.   2. Educational psychology.
3. Education, Humanistic.   I. Title.
Q181.S674   370.15   81-80241
ISBN 0-8022-2389-3   AACR2

Dedication

To Claudine, my wife, and mother of our six children: source of our strength, courage, and ideals.

Table of Contents

vii

viii

Preface

The idea of teaching holistically is not new. Sri Aurobindo wrote in 1910:

"The intellect is an organ composed of several groups of functions, divisible into two important classes, the functions and faculties of the right hand, the functions and faculties of the left. The faculties of the right hand are comprehensive, creative, and synthetic; the faculties of the left hand critical and analytic . . . the left limits itself to ascertained truth, the right grasps that which is still elusive or unascertained. Both are essential to the completeness of the human reason. These important functions of the machine have all to be raised to their highest and finest working-power, if the education of the child is not to be imperfect and onesided."[1]

With reference to the importance of teaching-learning in the affective domain, Eiss and Harbeck wrote:

"It is becoming increasingly apparent that the (affective domain) . . . has played a greater part in the learning process than most educators have been willing to admit. For example, there is evidence that increased awareness of facts of science often produces a dislike for science in many students, with the result that students avoid further learning situations.

"Probably a major factor in the failure to give adequate emphasis to affective goals is the difficulty of testing for their attainment . . . this has lead some educators to conclude that it is impossible to describe behaviors that would indicate the attainment of affective goals."[2]

The following model was proposed indicating assumed relationships of the three domains:

ix

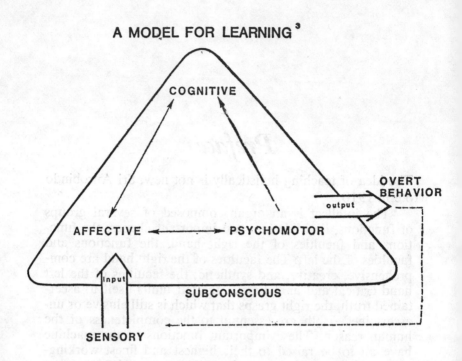

A MODEL FOR LEARNING [3]

COGNITIVE

AFFECTIVE ⟷ PSYCHOMOTOR

OVERT BEHAVIOR

output

Input

SUBCONSCIOUS

SENSORY

An attempt was made to relate the Eiss Model for Learning with the lateralized nature of the human brain—a prime factor of human development. Evidence is that the cognitive domain may be a function of the left hemispheric processes and that the affective domain may be a function of the right hemispheric processes. Yet stronger evidence indicates the equal and important roles of both hemispheres in the learning processes. Doran has expressed ". . . the fact that 'learning occurs holistically,' (through the three domains, and that) the last decade has urged upon us science instruction that is humanistic, individualized, value-oriented, as well as future-focused."[4]

To meet at least some of these demands, the model is altered thusly:

x

A MODEL FOR LEARNING WHICH DEMONSTRATES
THE ROLE OF BRAIN HEMISPHERICITY

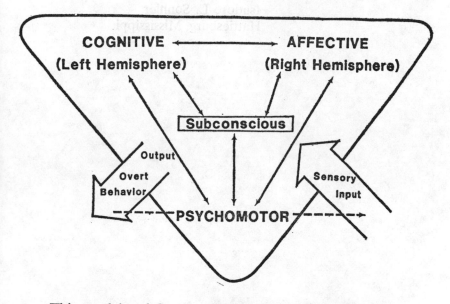

This model satisfies overwhelming evidence that affective and cognitive educational objectives should share desirable outcomes with equal effort. Further, it not only explains the nature of diversities among learners (and their teachers, as well), it justifies and lends credence to the need for their maintenance. It explains why educational systems (and their leaders) derive strength and gain degrees of effectiveness by not only maintaining, but catering to these human diversities.

Indeed, this kind of broadminded leadership yields unity and harmony— a very special kind of conformity. However, conformity, imposed for administrative convenience (by teacher, principal, or superintendent), enlivens these latent and potential diversities, creates disunity, and erodes the quality and effectiveness of that leadership.

To explain to *everyone* "how to provide educational leadership" is nearly an impossible task. Different people need different instructions. However, we did *"try to do it"* in this book and must apologize for those failures due to inevitable semantic barriers.

Isadore L. Sonnier
Hattiesburg, Mississippi

[1]Bogen, J. E. *The Human Brain* (Prentice Hall: Englewood Cliffs, N. J.) 1977, p. 134.

[2]Eiss, A. F. and M. B. Harbeck. *Behavioral Objectives in the Affective Domain* (National Science Teachers Association: Washington, D. C.) 1969, pp. 9-12.

[3]Eiss, A. F. Instructional Systems: Experimental *Edition* (National Science Teachers Association: Washington, D. C.) 1968, p. 25.

[4]Doran, R. L. *Basic Measurement and Evaluation of Science Instruction* (National Science Teachers Association: Washington, D.C.) 1980, preface, p. 1.

Acknowledgments

The author proudly acknowledges the assistance of the following teachers in locating other sources and bibliographic listings as well as in the editing of these materials. They are as follows:

Laura A. Alford
Coahoma High School
Clarksdale, Miss.

Linda C. Alford
Pine School
Franklinton, La.

Lynn Anderson
Poplarville Lower Elem.
Poplarville, Miss.

Patricia K. Brown
Kentwood Upper Elem.
Kentwood, La.

Sue S. Dennis
Morgantown Elem.
Natchez, Miss.

Diana Kay Derrick
Student, Univ. of So.
Miss.
Forest, Miss.

Ina Easterling
Ellisville Elementary
Ellisville, Miss.

Andy Lagarde
Pass Christian High
School
Pass Christian, Miss.

Martha Kaye Lowery
Ellisville Elementary
School
Ellisville, Miss.

Charlotte Mitchell
Ellisville Elementary
School
Ellisville, Miss.

Karen Myers
Poplarville Lower Elem.
School
Poplarville, Miss.

Mary Graves Pardes
Amite School Center
Liberty, Miss.

Lela V. Emmons
Schlater School
Schlater, Miss.

Doris F. Roland
Forest Elementary School
Forest, Miss.

John Curtis Harper
Prentiss Alternative
  School
Prentiss, Miss.

Sue Smith
Burnsville Elementary
  School
Burnsville, Miss.

Linda Keen
Raleigh Middle School
Raleigh, Miss.

Coe Alice Stirgus
Rocky Creek School
Lucedale, Miss.

The editorial comments of Dr. Robert T. Snyder are also acknowledged with this expression of appreciation and gratitude. And, without Karen Fletcher's typing and editing assistance, this project could have dragged on for months longer.

Introduction

PROVIDING LEADERSHIP

The following comments are offered as a general approach to educating students employing the teaching strategies which generally come under the heading of self-directed teaching (vs. authoritarian). So many persons have wanted to try these strategies, but were only offered disjointed advice or remnant solutions to its implementation.

Indeed, when discussing this work with educators throughout the country, the frequent comment was, "Everyone talks about doing these things in the classroom—educating both brain hemispheres, open education, humanistic education—but, I've seen little teaching in the affective domain; description of how to actually do it."

While this book is probably not able to completely communicate all of these qualities of education to all readers, it was attempted to give each person a sense of his own worth, his own philosophy, and an identity with actual pedagogies and classroom procedures.

While HOLISTIC EDUCATION applies universally in the affective teaching of any subject matter, it is especially discussed in these pages as having traits of humanistic education and open education with special emphases on human brain lateralization. The introduction opens the door to these strategies in educating students from early elementary to graduate school.

Leadership vs. Being in Charge

Being in charge does not necessarily mean that leadership is being provided. However, by providing leadership, you are definitely fulfilling your charge of responsibility to your students as a teacher.

The following suggestions are offered to assist teachers in assessing and/or improving their leadership qualities. The list is by no means an exclusive list. Nor is it intended to serve the needs of all teachers with the same degree of insight into themselves and their relations with their students. Hopefully, the scope is so broad and general that there should be something in it for everyone. These suggestions include:

1. *Help each person to play a role in ongoing classroom activities.*

Each student has a set of experiences that is unique to that person. Each student is capable not only of contributing, but of benefiting from group interactions. However, individual differences make some students more effective contributors than others. On the other hand, some students can actually benefit more from the contributions of others than if they were themselves contributing. Forced contributions can sometimes be devastating for some students. Others need the "confidence building" that classroom contributions foster. Not all students should be expected to gain the same degree of personal growth from any of your classroom activities or experience growth at the same rate.

2. *Provide opportunities for all students without regard to the "kind of person," "type of student," "grades earned," or any other form of discrimination.*

Not only is each person to play an active role in ongoing activities, but a very special effort should be made to insulate some students from being "type"-cast. It is relatively well established that a student's grade point average (often interpreted to be his scholastic abilities) has little or nothing to do with creativity.

Indeed, a number of investigators have found that if there is a relationship at all, the creative student is not the student that makes the best grades. Too, students that look intelligent are not necessarily the students that make the best grades. And, students that look intelligent may not be as intelligent as students that look dull.

Labels such as "intelligent" or "dull" are very subjective qualities and should be avoided like the plague. The teacher has clearly the responsibility to avoid being prejudiced in any way.

3. *Maintain high standards, but not at the expense of personal relations with students.*

This message is conveyed by the fact that you are a teacher of students, not an elementary school teacher, and not a teacher of social studies, mathematics or science. It is implied that if you teach students, they will relate to you better and, therefore, with what you are trying to teach.

If you are devoted to your subject, without regard to the needs of all of your students, only those with innate scholastic abilities learn. Scholastic abilities, as will be pointed out later, do not necessarily yield insight. Therefore you should temper cognitive objectives with affective objectives.

If you are rather authoritative in either the textbook or the lecture mode of teaching, or both, the students that benefit the most are those students that are more readily reached by such a presentation. Not all students learn well by reading and listening, even though those are the major skills necessary for "scholastic achievement" in our society.

Creative students do not do well, according to many authorities, if forced to learn by reading and listening to lectures. Neither should intelligence be equated with any degree of reading or listening skills.

For these and other reasons, it is MOST IMPORTANT to keep good relations with all of your students. It should be realized that there are few visible indicators telling of your success or failure to "teach," "reach," or "influence" students.

There are usually few indications of the impressions you create upon your students. A good rapport is merely a surface indicator. The students' enthusiasm goes a bit deeper. Ultimately, you should accept the fact that you can never reach "all" students "all the time."

The long range influence you have on students is even more difficult to predict. Therefore, you should expect the MOST out of all students and be receptive to THEIR BEST —their best by standards of mutual agreement.

4. *Emphasize the fact that the best learning environment is one in which the student is learning something with a personal investment—(the affective domain).*

This explains itself rather well. However, *how* to obtain this level of personal investment on the part of students is not that easy. The word is motivation, motivation and motivation. The following suggestions may be helpful in obtaining higher levels of personal investment in the classroom environment.

5. *Bring the group together often or regularly for interpersonal relations to account for their time and efforts.*

Science is "caught, not taught." So are enthusiasm, motivation and personal investment. These sessions are important and should be allowed to run their course. Do not push, pull or tug. Just allow students to talk about their successes, surprises, joys, disappointments and failures.

6. *Develop a freedom of discussion among students as well as among the students and yourself.*

Although this may sound easier said than done, in reality, each group is different. All groups need different degrees of motivation. Once started, some run on their own steam. Still other groups may be easily motivated, but tire very rapidly if left on their own.

This is where your skills as a facilitator will come in handy.

Be prepared to reward leadership and to avoid individuals (without total disregard) that take charge or accept responsibilities without knowing how to handle it. Leadership and followship qualities are in need of development in these individuals.

Those immediately ready to contribute really want to contribute. They may simply not know how. This is a reality that students themselves can detect and correct. Provide them with the opportunity for this to happen.

7. *Create an atmosphere of maximum team effort while at the same time holding each individual responsible and accountable for his own efforts.*

It is almost entirely due to leadership when students work well together. The quality of leadership provided will usually determine how well individual students are able to hold themselves accountable for the group as well as for their individual activities. It is not easy to "tell" another teacher how to achieve this degree of leadership. But one thing is certain. If all of these suggestions are followed, however, one will become a different kind of leader—a "facilitator."

8. *Provide an atmosphere of personal and interpersonal evaluations for the purpose of rewarding success or assisting with failures.*

While this point may seem to repeat the previous one, it is offered to assist in HOW to facilitate group interactions and team work. The key words are success and failure.

These extremes should occur without having negative reaction to failures. Failure may be nothing more than a temporary set-back. Students take a great deal of pride in helping one another out of these temporary set-backs. That, in itself, is a satisfying and motivating learning experience!

9. *Become a "facilitator" of the educational process in your classroom.*

Cause and allow activities to happen. Be the "good provider" of a suggestion, now and then. Provide that piece of equipment or material that may by its absence be preventing the forward progress of a group or an individual. By becoming a facilitator of the processes of science, you are also becoming a facilitator of a richly rewarding learning environment. Develop these skills in yourself as well as in your students.

Materials are provided in Part I to help you with the day-to-day plans as a facilitator. Students' materials are included. Part II explains *why* do it.

Part I

Students' Materials Basic Concepts: Sharing in How to Learn with Your Students

Chapter 1

The Two Faces of Science:
Knowledge and Processes

CONCEPTS

A. Science: The Body of Knowledge.
1. Knowledge catalogued into established disciplines, in the minds of men, for convenience of recall and data handling.
2. Knowledge yet to be learned is not catalogued.

B. Science: The Processes of Learning.
1. The acts and activities that assist us to gain new knowledge, among others, include:
   a. Counting
   b. Measuring
   c. Observing
   d. Data Gathering
   e. Data Processing
   f. Inferring
   g. Predicting

SKILLS AND PRINCIPLES

1. Identify the two faces of science and list their differences in the total picture of the scientific enterprise.

3

2. Identify their values in the classroom setting.
3. Identity needs for emphasizing science as a set of processes.
4. Know how the body of knowledge can be gained through the use of the set of processes.

Everyone knows *science as a body of knowledge*. According to that definition, what we DO in the science classroom is to learn more of the established bodies of scientific knowledge. The emphasis is on the *established knowledge*.

However, this is not all that science is. Nor should this be all that students gain from a science course. Because this definition is so widely accepted, the classroom setting usually plays far too great a role in the teaching and the learning of science. A rather "bookish" setting occurs.

On the other hand, science is like a two-sided coin. The flip side of the coin shows us *science as a set of processes*. These ARE the processes of learning. And, through these processes, we can (and should) equate science with learning —all learning and all disciplines.

The body of scientific knowledge is catalogued into the established disciplines—like chemistry, physics, biology, geology and even many others that are not normally considered science. These disciplines, of course, exist mostly in the minds of men.

According to some people, this is a terrible thing to say. But, for others, these disciplines are NOT REAL in the REAL WORLD. They are but tools for man's thinking. They exist for the convenience of data handling—cataloguing and recalling.

However, the processes of science assist us to learn the knowledge which is yet to be learned and catalogued. Indeed, that is WHAT the scientist DOES when he is the field and in the laboratory. He gathers and processes data. It can be observed that by this definition, not all scientists actively participate in the scientific enterprise.

The scientist counts, measures and observes things. He

4

orders, groups and classifies these data. Other processes that he performs include inferring and predicting, given a sufficient amount of data. There are many more of these processes that he performs from time to time, if he actively participates in the scientific enterprise.

While not so much on purpose, and sometimes rather haphazardly, scientists are trained in the use and application of the processes of science. A person who is a scientist almost has to have highly developed natural inclinations in the use and application of the processes of science. Because, in the minds of most scientists, a formal education in science means learning the body of knowledge of a discipline. However, informally, by trial and error, he learns HOW TO LEARN by using and applying the processes of science.

It is suggested that THE PROCESSES OF SCIENCE (the processes for discovering knowledge) be given more of an equal share of classroom time with SCIENCE: THE BODY OF KNOWLEDGE. By actively participating in data gathering activities, students can become proficient in the use and application of the processes of science.

Students should be taught these processes. However, it has been said that SCIENCE IS MORE CAUGHT THAN TAUGHT. Even so, it should not be left to chance that individuals with the proper natural inclinations will enter into the scientific enterprise. THE SCIENTIFIC ENTERPRISE IS FOR EVERYONE!

A reporter, sifting out a story, uncovers it with the processes of science. So does the historian in the task of determining how an event of the past really happened.

Actually, this is the BEST TRAINING we can give our so-called non-science students. The term "so-called" is used because non-science students need the processes of science proficiency as well as do the science students. And, who knows how many children, naturally inclined in the use of these processes, we have failed to reach because of this mismanagement and/or misunderstanding?

5

For the Teacher:

The question that some students and teachers alike may ask at this point is, what happens to the learning of the body of knowledge while students are dabbling with the process? Simply, the evidence is that they gain MORE OF THE BODY OF KNOWLEDGE as well as to gain a HEALTHIER ATTITUDE AND CURIOSITY about SCIENCE IN GENERAL, although, the amount of knowledge gained may have to be sacrificed for the latter. The cognitive domain is tempered with the affective domain.

When one realizes HOW SCIENCE IS LEARNED, the processes of science become even more of an attractive tool of education. *Learning science is often the converging of ideas that one has already observed and knows.*

However, the larger concepts are hardly ever put together in the classroom. They come to us when walking, driving, when sitting quietly or in the roar of a football stadium. When we least expect it, the larger concepts of science come to us like turning on a light—often like a bolt of lightning.

The general understanding of science, as processes, very likely must be discussed by you with your students. It is not likely that they will come to grips with these sophisticated concepts without verbal communication. However, verbal communication being what it is, ineffective and a poor way of communicating, these concepts will have to be placed before the students time and time again—especially after a pleasant learning experience.

Come back to discussions of the two faces of science after students have gathered and processed data. They will have an even greater need to see science this way at that time. It will make everything else they're doing fall into understandable place.

6

Chapter 2

How to Select a Topic

CONCEPTS

A. Must be one of interest to student.
B. Must relate with student's own curiosity.
C. Uncovering information should be exciting and increase student's desire to uncover further.

SKILLS AND PRINCIPLES

A. The motivation level that a student has toward his own topic will determine his interest and the amount of time he is willing to spend uncovering information.
   1. Time spent in classroom discussions, allowing individuals to express interest (or disinterest) in topics, is well worth the effort. REGROUP, DISCUSS FURTHER, if necessary.
   2. Objective of classroom discussions is for individuals to separate into smaller and smaller groups, sending them away knowing WHAT to do and HOW to do it.
B. Monitor student efforts during the compilation phase of their project toward the objective that individuals continue to relate toward the culmination of their project.
C. A well selected topic, in an atmosphere of general group interest, increases the individual's desire to

7

explore further. The more that is uncovered, the greater the desire to uncover further.

For the Teacher:

The selection of a unit of study is one of the most important tasks in the art of teaching. Topic ideas could come from a number of sources. The time-honored source for curriculum direction is the textbook. Many textbooks offer an excellent diving board into student-centered learning experiences.

HOW TO DIRECT the upcoming unit is the next question. You have the option of presenting the materials in the traditional, teacher-centered manner. Or, you may already be teaching through student initiative and their resources. You may already be a student-centered teacher.

These ideas are offered to assist those teachers who would like to allow their students to guide themselves through their own learning experiences. Textbooks and current events are among the most fertile grounds for identifying topics for a student-centered unit of study.

In either case, these are the signs of a successful unit of study: 1) The subject matter is well covered, 2) The enthusiasm level is held high, 3) Individuals gain healthy attitudes toward learning.

Indeed, sometimes the students enjoy learning so much that they don't believe that they are learning anything. After all, learning is supposed to be a difficult, dragging, and painful experience. It would not serve your public relations profile well for this belief to go beyond your classroom. Make your students aware of the volumes of materials that they have uncovered and shared with each other.

A Student-Centered Unit Is an Expression of "Open" Education. There are probably as many ways of opening the curriculum to students as there are student-centered teachers. However, there are probably a number of common strings running through all of these (curriculum) open classrooms.

In opening up a textbook unit, one way to get students

8

started is to establish the boundaries: Unit II, Chapters 12 through 15, just Chapter 12, or just one of the sections in a given chapter.

Once the boundaries are set, have students scan the ideas that are at hand—those presented in the textbook. "What are we going to be studying next?" Have them talk about it. "Is anyone familiar with these topics already?" "Where else could we gather information concerning these topics?" A healthy discussion, at this point, assures you of a well-received unit of work.

A mum class assures you of failure. Failure could come for several reasons: 1) Not enough timely-interest; 2) students are insufficiently motivated; 3) you are, yourself, lacking the spirit of these teaching strategies; or 4) you don't know the subject matter sufficiently to transmit this security into the group, among others.

The motivation level that a student has toward his own topic will determine his interest and the amount of time he is willing to spend uncovering information.

During the first round of discussions, list topics that students suggest for further study. A chalkboard list will have the unifying effect of one unit of study and the diverging effect of causing individuals to express interests and personal commitments toward individual components of the total unit.

Time spent in these classroom discussions is well worth the effort. Allow individuals to express their interests (or disinterests) in the individual topics or the unit, itself; therefore, have students GROUP and REGROUP and discuss further, if necessary.

The prime objective of these discussions is to separate and segregate individuals each towards his own personal commitment with a topic for his own project. The ideal is to have a topic covered by a group of four or five students—probably no more than six. Then, have each individual act rather possessive toward uncovering information on subtopics of this larger topic. Start the information-gathering process.

Monitor student efforts during this compilation phase of the unit. A student that is not progressing well could well be compared with the rotten apple in a barrel. He will get others involved in his non-related activities (better referred to as a potential discipline problem). The student doesn't want this anymore than you do. He may like to be the "Visual Aide Director" for his group—surely, you'll think of something!

The prime objective at this point is that individuals continue to relate toward the culmination of their projects. In most cases, minor alterations will have to be made—expanding their topics to include a newspaper article found here or there, for example. In a few cases, a major alteration will have to be made. Select a new topic, trade with another student toward mutual satisfaction, or find a totally different task for an individual: 1) Help another class member with teaching aids; 2) Help locate materials that any class member needs as a teaching aid; 3) Help explore possibilities for the next unit that the class is to study, etc.

Generally speaking, a well selected topic, in an atmosphere of group interest, increases the individual's desire to explore further. The enthusiasm is "catching." Too, the more that is uncovered, the greater the desire to uncover further.

Comments to Share with Students:

Everyone has things in which they are interested. Such interests are a natural outgrowth of a healthy and happy individual. They range from a burning curiosity to a lukewarm desire to know something. The things that interest us vary greatly from person to person.

However, we tend to get excited when we find someone who likes the things that we like. Our best friends are those persons with whom we like to discuss these interests. The things we have in common with one another add to the quality of our friendships and to the quality of our lives in general.

That is the purpose of this lesson. Although we will actually use examples in the science, this procedure could be used in any other of our classes. The procedure is simple, but it produces excellent results.

It calls for each person to lend himself to the situation

and share his knowledge and experiences with others in his group. Each one will have to express his likes and dislikes, his feelings, as well as what he knows and what he would like to know. The "group contributions" must truly be a representation of everyone in the group.

The purpose of the early group meetings is to establish a number of topics to be studied by the class. As these topics are refined and assigned to individuals, group meetings are conducted for the purpose of accommodating each individual with his own personal project, or, individual topic.

These topics could come out of the textbook you are studying or they could come from current events. The only thing of importance is that each student have a personal commitment toward the selection of the topic to be studied and that he have at least some interest in a small portion of the overall unit.

Don't hesitate to volunteer for a "new" topic about which you would like to know more. You won't stand alone. There will be others to have similar topics. You will want to share materials you find with them and others can do the same for for you. Each person should support and cooperate with each other.

In order for you to get the most satisfaction from the work that you are doing, there must be a growing curiosity into the topic—the more you find, the more interested you get in your project. It is important that you have this sort of devotion to your project.

Anything less than this enthusiasm could cause you to lose interest in the topic you are uncovering. If this happens, this should be shared with your other group members and your teacher. First, the group may have a member willing to trade topics with you. If so, this may take care of the problem.

Second, the teacher may know of someone else, in another group, with whom you may wish to swap topics. Most probably, the teacher will wish to help you as you make the transition from one topic to another. Actually, the work you have done thus far on the first topic should be helpful toward making the decisions concerning your next topic.

11

Chapter 3

Where to Find Information

CONCEPTS

A. Real problems have a way of being all-consuming in time, effort and a challenge to one's ability to uncover information.

B. The problem will tell you how to handle itself.
1. The type of data needed will determine where to get them.
2. The type of data you receive or uncover will tell you how it should be handled.

SKILLS AND PRINCIPLES

A. Provide time for students to obtain information wherever and whenever they have a need to get it.

B. Recognize the difference between the use of the textbook as a tool for learning vs. the use of library resources with the textbook being one of these resources.

C. Experiment with the values of textbook problems vs. real problems (which do not preclude the use of textbooks) in learning environments.

D. Equate the flow of information in your classroom with flow of data and help your students to see themselves processing data.

For the Teacher:

If students are to be sufficiently prepared to teach the class

12

through their own initiative and their own resources, they will have to be provided with a sufficient amount of time to collect the necessary information.

You have allowed individuals to group and to regroup towards the objective that each person ends up knowing WHAT he is to do and HOW he is to do it. They have all selected a topic of interest to themselves and towards the satisfaction of a larger group topic.

The next question you ask is where to find this information. What to do with 30 or 35 students—each with a grand plan for learning something about his own special problem. Recognize the difference between the use of the textbook as a tool for learning and the use of the library—books, in general— with the textbook being just another resource book.

Have your students be aware of the people in their community that can and would be willing helpers toward the completion of their project. Besides the school library, there are usually public libraries available. And, there may be a museum that the entire class can go to for a specific lesson or for general enrichment.

Think of PEOPLE, PLACES AND THINGS as resources. There may be factories and industries in the community with "people" resources, or with guided tours for the specific or general enrichment of study plans. Let the students make the original contacts. Some can follow through to the end —others will need your support and assistance. It goes without saying that the school administrators will also need to be involved before the finalizing of any of these plans.

Aside from these resources of information, there is one potential which is well worth your attention. Practically any project you do, or the students do, can be made into a "real problem" or a "real experience" for your students. Real problems have a way of requiring interdisciplinary thinking for their solution. Too, they have a way of being very fertile "curriculum" materials.

If your problem leads to it, call for resource persons from the community to assist your students. Let one thing lead to another—without getting out of hand, of course.

13

Recognizably, the flow of information may get out of control. So, if you see your task as processing data, it may make a little more sense and be helpful in keeping everything under control. Every piece of information that flows from outside the classroom into the classroom can be thought of as being a datum. All this data must be processed.

Consider even the biography of one of your guest speakers as data. Someone will have to collect it and it will have to be dispensed at a particular time and place. All data will have to be collected from the world, processed, and at a specific time be dispensed in the classroom as a learning experience.

A good communication system, such as a posted list of "who is doing what topic," can be a helpful tool in the processing of data. When one student runs across some information which is clearly John's or Susan's, he will proudly share it with the right person.

In essence, an important factor in data collection is that most data you find, or collect, will tell you what to do with it itself. You immediately know that you can or cannot use it. You immediately know that you will need to get more like this one, or that one. Or you know that it belongs to one of the other students.

The whole point of this data collection phase is for the purpose of sharing with the other students as a culminating activity of this entire process. Therefore, while you could be called a student-centered teacher, you should also think of yourself as a facilitator of the educational process—making it happen.

Comments for Students:

Practically any project you select for sharing with the class can be made into a "real problem," or a "real experience." This could well be the pointer that heads you in the right direction: For just about any subject you are studying, somewhere, there is someone who makes a living "doing" the things that you are "studying." Your job? Find him.

14

Find that person and speak with him. What are the special things that he has to know in order to do his work? Where can one get this kind of training? Start with *people*. Then, think of *places* and *things*.

When you think of places to find information, libraries immediately come to mind. Start with your own school library and some home libraries. Places also include museums. Many museums have libraries and some even have speakers that would either speak with your class in the museum or in your classroom.

Think of THINGS like factories and the various industries in your community. They, too, like to relate with students. However, you should always clear with your teacher any of these arrangements PRIOR to your making them.

Remember to make "real problems" from your *people, places and things* involvements. *Make in the classroom* some of the things that they manufacture. Involve as many of the class members in your project as you possibly can. The nice thing about being involved is that "involvement usually calls for having to know something before you can get involved." Learning usually has to take place. So too with real problems in which you will get involved.

Group planning, of the nature you would do in the classroom, calls for collecting and shuffling data and information from person to person—some acting on the information and others passing it on. Think of and call this information "data." You will need data in order to conduct a class field trip. You will want to collect data pertaining to the guest speakers you will invite to your class.

The flow of this data from "outside the classroom" to "inside the classroom" and to all individuals will need some processing. THE PROBLEM WILL TELL YOU HOW TO HANDLE IT ITSELF. Discuss with the responsible individuals, or the committee, the needed data. Determine what information WILL BE needed.

Once you know what is needed, GO AFTER THE INFORMATION. WHAT IS NEEDED will tell you WHERE TO

15

GET IT. If you are collecting information on a report you are to make to the class, it is quickly obvious that you are to go to PEOPLE (experts in the community who can serve as resource persons), PLACES OR THINGS (laboratories, libraries, museums, factories, etc.).

Once you start obtaining information, or data, it should be obvious to you that it is garbled. You can use some and some you simply cannot use. Some will be handy for a class-mate, but not for you. Some of which you will consider important while others are of lesser importance.

Some data you will receive will tell you that you need more like it. The simple message of all this is that THE TYPE OF DATA YOU RECEIVE WILL TELL YOU HOW IT SHOULD BE HANDLED. You will immediately know that this is YOUR data, or JOHN'S or SUSAN's data.

If John and Susan, and the rest of the class feel the same need to collect and share information, everyone prospers. Everyone is collecting data of a particular kind (John: hurricanes and Susan: tornadoes, for example). The overall purpose is that John, Susan, and others, will be sharing this information with the class in the near future.

Chapter 4

Conducting an Experiment

CONCEPTS

A. All things being equal: Variables.
   1. Control group—A normal (or usual) situation or condition.
   2. Experimental Group—The group which receives the "different" treatment or treatments (one at the time). Or it is the new idea which is being tried out.
   3. Age, sex and other differences within groups.

B. The experiment performed, should be repeatable by someone else, and they should get the same data originally gotten—or similar data.
   1. To be kept in mind when establishing a treatment design.
   2. To be kept in mind when describing the experiment—leaving no doubt in the mind of the reader as to how to repeat the experiment.

SKILLS AND PRINCIPLES

1. All things being equal, variables are tested one at a time.
2. A control group establishes the normality of the situation.
3. Experimental groups establish the difference or results

17

from having applied variable situations or conditions.

4. An investigation has been well conceived, initiated, and reported when it can be repeated in its entirety and similar results obtained.

Comments for Students:

From time to time there comes the need for learning if this product is better than that one or if this procedure is superior to that one. A controlled experiment can be so structured that it will assist in the determination of the best product or procedure. The results of a controlled experiment usually make good science fair projects, displaying the results and describing the procedures of the experiment.

To conduct a controlled experiment is really to test one thing against another. A race is a controlled experiment. All runners are made to undergo a common course. They are all started at the same time. In other words, EVERYTHING is equal for all contestants—except for the variables which are each relative: 1) strength, 2) endurance, 3) speed, and a number of others such as length of stride and muscular coordination for that particular event.

So with a scientific experiment. To test the best of several products of a particular grocery item, they are all made to perform a number of tests. Usually, each product gains its own set of superior ratings for some of the tests while showing a poor performance on other tests. The idea is to pick the MOST CONSISTENTLY high or superior-performing product.

If breakfast cereals were being tested for the opposite feature of sogginess vs crunchiness, the results could be subjective (a matter of opinion). Some persons would give a cereal superior rating for being soggy while others would rate the crunchy one superior. Consequently, it should be recognized when collecting data that there could be a variable quality within one of the variables to be tested.

When you decide what it is that you want to test, set up all of the qualities that are to be tested—your variables.

When you have decided that you will pit all of these qualities against each other, one at a time, you have constructed your research design. And, you are ready to start the data collection process.

Catalog your data for each product, by trials, and by variable. Or, catalog each test for each variable for each individual thing being tested against each other.

Often the simplest data is the best. For example, by ranking each cereal first through fifth for the five cereals being investigated is a good way. That way, $1 = $ low and $5 = $ high would yield the largest number of points to indicate superior quality and the lowest number of points to indicate lower quality, keeping in mind the possible subjectivity of some of the variables.

The problem of subjective variables can be eliminated if in the design it is worked out to determine how many persons call one quality superior and how many call the other quality superior. Then merely report the findings.

Chapter 5

Gathering Data

CONCEPTS

A. Controversial issues yield more diverse (better) data.
B. Designing a method for gathering the data (research design).
C. Constructing an instrument.
D. Applying the instrument, the nature of the group studied.
E. The size of the population and its randomness.

SKILLS AND PRINCIPLES

1. How to select a data gathering project.
2. How to design an instrument with which to gather the data.
3. How to apply an instrument for best results, representative and random sampling.
4. What constitutes good and reliable data.

Comments for Students:

The nature of the project you select will have much to do with the data you are able to collect from it. A more controversial issue will yield more diverse data than will a bland topic that is not even an issue in the minds of different people.

20

Therefore, for your first real problem or investigation, you should pick a topic about which people argue. It will make the difference between trying to process bland data (everyone answered all of the questions the same way) and "good" or "better" data.

The term "good" data generally means that the data accurately describes what they are supposed to describe. Good data means accurate and useful information. The term "better" is generally applied to data with a wide range of information, the opposite of bland data.

Once you have selected your topic or issue, determine the questions that you can ask to find out the things you will want to know about the topic or issue. What questions can you ask that will separate the different ways that people feel about the issue? Start with the BIG QUESTION. "Are you FOR ....?" Chapters 6 and 7 discuss the construction of various kinds of instruments.

Once the instrument is constructed, try it out on a small population. Such a *pilot study* can often yield some real sore spots in the instrument—if not some real problems with the entire project! Probably the most important question to ask about your instrument at this point is, "Does it do what it is supposed to do?"

If it does, the next step is to determine the population to which it can best be applied in order to get the best data. Since most populations number in the hundreds and thousands, it is obvious that you cannot allow EACH PERSON in the overall (total) population to participate in your project. So, determine WHO or WHAT constitutes the overall or TOTAL population.

Is it to be the union of all "students" in your school? Your town? State? Once you have determined the inclusive population, determine a way in which to actually contact just a small "representative" portion or "sample" of this population.

You cannot reach each person in your population. Even if the sample is small enough—like a small school with about

21

100 students, you do not want to sample the entire population. However, you will want a representative sample which is RANDOMLY SELECTED—a "random sample" to represent the entire population.

Randomness means that everyone in the population HAD THE OPPORTUNITY to participate. Everyone COULD HAVE participated—had they been at the right place at the right time. However, only a small, representative sample could physically be handled.

A random sample can be obtained on purpose. That could be done by going to each home room and picking out the first two or three persons on the teacher's roll book. Or, a list of all students drawn out of a hat is a random sample.

You can chance a random selection for your sample. The first 30 to arrive at school in the morning could be acceptable as a random sample of your student body. Or, 10 students in each of three lunchroom, P.E., or recess periods in which all students participate. Be sure to work out the students that do not participate in these "regular school events" and report this discrepancy in your data.

For example, you obtained your random sample of your community from the phone book. And, you will apply a telephone interview as your instrument. Realize that if 10 percent of your community's population does not have a phone, or is not listed in the phone book, YOUR DATA CAN ONLY BE ACCURATE TO THE POSSIBILITY OF A 10 PERCENT ERROR.

This sample has the potential of a 10 percent error in the data that you obtain from it. Realize, too, that a 10 percent error in most circumstances can be considered as very fine and reliable data. Any action you take on the recommendation of 90 percent of a population could and should be considered okay to do.

Every motorist in your area can be sampled at one of your busy street corners. However, the population will also include the rest of your county, state, and the United States. A sample of the license plates will tell you that.

Therefore, you may wish to find out how many passengers, on the average, are being transported in each vehicle with respect to the origin of the vehicle. Such a study, or survey, would tell you, among other things, 1) kind of vehicle, 2) its origin, 3) number of passengers—to be broken down by a) males, b) females, c) adults, and d) children. What else could you learn from this study?

Your biology teacher has several thousand fruit flies in a net cage. If you wish, you could simply reach in and capture approximately thirty: a) all at one time, or b) over a period of several weeks or months as you study one at a time. Would either of these collection methods be "good" sampling techniques?

The first method would be acceptable if the thirty flies were gathered with equal representation from the center and the eight corners (or throughout all areas of the cage). The second method could also have problems. The samples cut across several generations of flies. And, if each generation is changing one of its characteristics, at least with that characteristic, your data would be garbled.

However, if you had collected all thirty files on each of several monthly samples and analyzed each, you MAY be able to catch this change. Each sample may differ only slightly from one sample to the other. However, there would be a wide range of differences from the first to the last, several months apart.

It can be fun to collect and process data so as to find things out. However, the task can get out of hand. It has to be planned from start to finish. All along the way, you will have to establish the rules of the game. Mostly, it is a matter of keeping the project neat, simple, and within your limited time and physical abilities.

23

Chapter 6

An Instrument: The Questionnaire

CONCEPTS

A. Determining the population MOST SUITED to yield the data desired.
B. Developing an instrument which will yield the data desired.
C. Applying an instrument.
D. Processing data.

SKILLS AND PRINCIPLES

1. What instruments are.
2. The questionnaire as a data-gathering instrument.
3. The use of variables on a data-gathering instrument.
4. The construction of a questionnaire.
5. Constructing a questionnaire for a) convenience of participants, b) clear communications, and c) ease of processing the data.
6. Applying numerical values to common responses.
7. Printed or handed-out questionnaires (as a survey instrument) should not exceed ten items.

Comments for Students:

Instruments are the extensions of our senses. They help us in performing our everyday tasks. Another term that is used is "a tool." The microscope takes us into the micro-

24

cosmos while the telescope lets us see the macrocosmos, just to name two of the instruments of science.

The screwdriver is designed to achieve a task that one's fingernail just could not accomplish (although most of us can remember breaking a fingernail that way). With the right instrument, work is accomplished with so much more ease.

Another task in science is to collect data. A tool or instrument can be devised to dig into the minds of men, without changing their opinions, and determine exactly the nature of these opinions. The questionnaire is just such an instrument. One can be devised to determine (ahead of time and without changing the minds of the men sampled) how an upcoming election will end up, the size of a population in favor of or against abortion, the equal rights amendment, or a simple question such as how many parents would support a movement to air condition a school.

Schools keep records on all students. The way that they get the information is by having parents fill out questionnaires. They are asked your age, birthday, sex, height, weight, illness, and something about brothers and sisters.

In your record are such data as your letter grades for each subject of each grade level, your attendance records, awards, and sometimes comments of teachers. From folder to folder, there are these kinds of data for each student, most of which were obtained by way of instruments.

One kind of instrument is the questionnaire. From this instrument you can find out how your fellow students would vote in a presidential, gubernatorial, or mayoral race. You can find how they feel about abortion or any of the social issues of the times. So, LET'S DO IT.

You will first want to construct your instrument. The instrument will be applied as a printed sheet that can be checked or easily filled in, starting with the variables such as male-female, age, student or non-student, religion, political party, and any other variable that is actually needed. DO NOT PUT VARIABLES on your instrument just for the sake of putting them on. Ask only those that are needed in order to process the given data.

25

Below the variables, determine the ordered set of questions that you will be asking. Start with THE BIG ONE: "1. If you were a registered voter, you would register as a Democrat .... Republican........ Independent........ Other....................
2. If you could vote in the upcoming election, for whom would you cast your presidential (other) vote?..............................
Questions 3 through 8 or 10 could ask if these are the same expressions as that of their parents, who influence them most—parents, teachers, or school mates, and other questions, such as: Should people be made to pay to cast their votes?

In most cases, ask the first question—which leads to the second, on until the topic is exhausted—*not to exceed ten questions for a printed questionaire.* (If the topic cannot be exhausted under ten questions, revise the instrument until that limitation can be met.)

A Pitfall. Be careful NOT TO ASK in the same question, "Are you *for* or *against* the passing of the school bond?" This really is two questions. You have no way of knowing if the response of "yes" means "yes I am for" or "yes, I am against" it.

Ways of Responding to Your Questions. First, you want to make it easy for them to answer. Second, you want their answers to be easily tabulated and analyzed. So you can accomplish this by providing, at the end of each question, Yes........ No........ Undecided........ Rarely there may be an instrument that must be answered yes or no without an undecided response. However, this should be the execption and not the rule. ALWAYS give a person the right to be undecided. Sometimes, this response will be an important one.

"Undecided" becomes an important response if you will treat all data on a scale of "1 through 3," like this: $1 = $ No, $2 = $ Undecided, and $3 = $ Yes. That gives you all shades between 1 and 3 with 2 being the *neutral middle,* 1 being no or *never,* and 3 being *yes or always.*

If a number system is used, consider 1 through 5 instead of 1 through 3. In this range, $1 = $ no/never, $3 = $ undecided, $5 = $ yes/always. On your questionnaire, write this:

26

EXAMPLE: (Circle 1 = no/never, 3 = undecided, 5 = yes/always)
1. Are you for the passing of the school bond?

1   2   3   4   5

(Again, remember the pitfall and do not ask both, "are you for or against," in the same question. You would not know if a 1 means "no, I am for" or "no, I am against.")

Although Chapter 8 is written to assist you with your data processing, a couple of pointers could be made here. A partially filled questionnaire should not be used unless the information ACTUALLY GIVEN is helpful. If participants write in reasons for responding the way that they do, let this be a clue that you have probably omitted a question that needed to be included on the questionnaire before this point. And you should have caught this mistake in your pilot study.

The Art of Instrument Building. The constructing of instruments is an art which can be developed by anyone. It is commonly practiced to build a four- or five-page instrument which will hopefully leave no stone unturned in its reliability. (RELIABILITY of an instrument is its abilty to obtain the desired information with thoroughness and accuracy each time. VALIDITY of an instrument is its ability to consistently obtain reliable data when applied for a particular purpose, circumstance, or condition.)

With the help of a computer, these data are processed and analyzed for differences and relationships (multiple regression) that each item has with each of the other items for each variable.

THIS IS ONE WAY to get good and reliable data. However, it is asking a lot of the population sampled to spend that much time out of a busy schedule to respond properly (four or five pages!). Indeed, this practice has built-in limitations: 1) The busiest individuals simply do not respond. 2) Those that do respond reach a tiring point, or boredom, and

27

haphazardly respond—lowering the degree of reliability and possibly validity.

IT IS MORE SKILLFUL to go after the desired data with the purpose and intent of retrieving just what you need—no more, no less. To do so is like placing a target on the side of a barn wall. Then you shoot just at the target. To do the opposite is like scattering shots at the entire side of the barn. The target being in the middle, it gets a fair share of shots.

Validating an Instrument. To simplify what could be a complicated activity, validating an instrument simply means that you go to others, familiar with the activity, and seek their opinion as to the fact that each item of your instrument does what it was designed to do.

Call those other persons a *panel of judges.* With either a brief oral or written statement from you, they are to know the general nature of your investigation. Then, on a checklist, they should check "yes........ no........ undecided........" as to whether each item will accurately obtain the desired data.

ALL instruments MUST be validated. And, the validating procedures and results are as much a necessary part of the investigation as any of the other activities. They too will have to be described in the final report.

Chapter 7

An Instrument: The Interview

CONCEPTS

A. Instruments are the extensions of our senses, aids in task-performance.
B. The interview is a commonly used instrument for collecting data.
C. Determine the population best suited to yield the desired data.
D. Develop the instrument that will yield the desired data.
E. Apply the instrument.

SKILLS AND PRINCIPLES

1. The interview is one of the most commonly applied data-gathering instruments.
2. How to develop an interview instrument.
3. How to apply an interview instrument.
4. The telephone lends itself to a deeper application of the interview instrument.
5. A limitation of the interview instrument is that time is a limiting factor to the quantity of data accessible.
6. Oral interviews should not exceed five items.

Comments for Students:

One of the most commonly used instruments is the inter-

29

view. Granted, most persons who are performing an interview don't know that they are applying such an instrument. The dentist's secretary was interviewing you when she was filling in the chart from the questions she asked you.

Any time someone needs to know something from you and asks the appropriate question to find it out, you are being interviewed. The form onto which the information is written is "the instrument" and the method for obtaining the information is "the interview."

If you decide that the interview is the way to collect the information you need, proceed in this manner. You should, by now, have your topic or issue established. Several questions will have to be settled, each helping to organize or to contribute to each other: WHAT will you be asking on the instrument and WHO will participate are of immediate concern. Remember that the telephone lends itself towards a deeper application of the interview instrument.

Developing Your Instrument. Realize that when you are interviewing a person, you have but a few seconds to complete the data-gathering task. That's all that MOST PERSONS can afford to give you. Therefore, try to get from them all of the information you will need in just a few questions— like five questions, for example.

Ask the biggest question first. Are you for the passing of the school bond? Or are you for the Equal Rights Amendment? Or for the freedom of women to have abortions with public funds? Your questionnaire will not assume these are right or wrong—but merely will determine how males feel about it, females, young adults, older adults, middle-aged, etc.

Ask an ordered set of questions. The first item (or question) of your instrument should be broad and general so as to place the participants' thoughts onto your topic. The first question leads to the next, and the next, *until the topic is exhausted— not to exceed five questions for an oral interview*. If the interview instrument does not exhaust the topic in five questions, revise it until it does.

Try the instrument out on some friends, on your class. Process the data. This pilot study should bring out some sore

30

spots about your instrument and the project, in general. This is your last opportunity to sharpen the instrument (and its ability to yield good data). Is the instrument discriminating? Do different persons answer it differently—males like other males and females like other females? If so, your instrument will yield good data and you have a good project.

Yes, no and undecided (I don't know) answers should be expected. If your participant feels that he should make a statement qualifying why he has answered "yes" or "no," revise the instrument until a definite "yes" or "no" and undecided position is clearly responded.

Data sheets, prepared in advance, are helpful in both collecting data and processing it later. Write in a check-list form for any and all variables needed for this project. Do not call for variables that you do not need.

Applying the Instrument. The instrument is developed and you know that you will be seeking about thirty participants. Know your age-level cut-offs, if it applies—only teenagers, only adults over twenty-one, all ages, etc. When seeking the assistance of a person to participate in your project, you will want to seek his permission. Ask the person if he/she has time to answer a few questions. State the nature of your project (BRIEFLY!!!), PAUSE, then begin with ITEM ONE of your instrument.

As you are completing the final question (face-to-face interview), jot down the appropriate information (which can be obtained by the physical appearance of the participant): Male........ Female........; Approximate Age.......; Married .... Single........; Blonde........ Brunnette........ Red Hair........; or any other physical feature that is needed in order to process the data by the variables selected.

Data is data and it all looks the same almost without regard to its origin. Therefore, make reference to Chapter VIII at this point concerning the processing of the data you have obtained from these interviews.

Chapter 8

Data Processing

CONCEPTS

A. Tally sub-groups in the various dichotomies.
B. Tally all questions by dichotomies.
C. These figures are RAW DATA.
D. Convert raw data into REFINED DATA: percentages, graphs, charts, tables, etc.
E. Data is refined for the purpose of making comparisons from dichotomy to dichotomy and from variable to variable.

SKILLS AND PRINCIPLES

1. A well-constructed instrument lends itself to ease in processing the data.
2. Collecting data on tabulation forms will add to the ease of describing or reporting the data.
3. Changing raw data into refined data.
4. Displaying data by use of visual aids.

Comments for Students:

When constructing an instrument, have the foresight to make data processing easier. Data processing is always difficult and tedious. However, it can be made easier and less time consuming. At the same time, the data can be so precise as to

32

describe EXACTLY the phenomenon it was designed to describe.

Oral or written questionnaires are discussed. However, these explanations could apply to many other data-gathering projects. Probably the easiest way to process these kinds of data is to simply pile the questionnaires up by variables—start with the male/female parameter. Place all sheets marked "male" on one stack and those marked "female" on another stack.

Break this down further: All "males, Grade 6" on one stack, "males, Grade 7" on another, and "males, Grade 8" in another stack. Do the same for all of the female sheets. All of these can be broken down further—all that "bring their own lunch" and all that "eat in the lunchroom."

Now, tally on a large tabular scoreboard with all of the categories provided for (see Table I, Sample Data Tabulation Form). Note that the result of these tabulations is a *histogram*. Your raw data has now been refined. The histogram so refines your data as to show you a picture of which item has more and which has fewer participants.

TABLE 1

SAMPLE DATA TABULATION FORM

			1	2	3	4	5	6	7	8	9	10	11	12	13	14	15
	GRADE 6	OWN LUNCH															
	N=_____	LUNCHROOM															
MALES	GRADE 7	OWN LUNCH															
N=___	N=_____	LUNCHROOM															
	GRADE 8	OWN LUNCH															
	N=_____	LUNCHROOM															
	GRADE 6	OWN LUNCH															
	N=_____	LUNCHROOM															
FEMALES	GRADE 7	OWN LUNCH															
N=___	N=_____	LUNCHROOM															
	GRADE 8	OWN LUNCH															
	N=_____	LUNCHROOM															

33

More important, from this chart, you can calculate the percentages for each category. Divide the totals into the subtotals after adding two decimal positions to the right. In other words, all percentage expressions have 100 as their common denominators. The significance of this will be pointed out in Chapter 9, Reporting the Findings.

Simply stated, the task at hand in data processing is to convert disjointed information, a little bit of it on each participants's sheet, into something manageable and understandable.

However, once you have tallied all of these results, you still have RAW DATA. It must be REFINED into information that is clearly understood and that can be compared from one question to the other. This is done by the use of percentages, graphs, charts, diagrams and visual aids of any kind. It is always helpful to display data by using visual aids.

Once the data is so simplified as to be called refined, the next task is to describe the results—or write up the results. Think of your project as having tossed up a bunch of numbered or colored chips. They fall to the ground. Now your task is to describe the relationships that each chip has with the others. Another expression is "leave no stone unturned." In other words, describe thoroughly and completely the results that you have obtained (see Chapter 9, Reporting the Findings).

Chapter 9

Reporting the Findings

CONCEPTS

A. The value of reporting in refined data rather than in rough data.
B. The value of visual aids to accompany refined data.
C. The text of a report.

SKILLS AND PRINCIPLES

1. Generally speaking, all reports of scientific investigations have a common format: a) the project discussed, b) procedure, c) results, and d) conclusions.
2. The project discussed includes the introduction, hypotheses, statements, and sometimes a project justification.
3. The review of the literature has its greatest advantage in being a credit to the researcher and an indication of his maturity, expertise, and competence.
4. The procedure section discusses the instrument, its application, data treatment, and the population or quality sampled.
5. Discuss results in simple language as though you were telling it to a friend (placing the exact data or results in parentheses).
6. The conclusions, like the introduction, are dedicated to the researcher and his involvement with the project or topic.

35

Comments for Students:

A project worth doing is a project worth reporting. Someone somewhere is interested in the results of your project. Generally speaking, all reports of scientific investigations have a common format: 1) The Project Discussed, 2) Procedure, 3) Results, and 4) Conclusions.

1) *The Project Discussed.* The discussion of a project generally starts with an *introduction*. *Hypotheses* are stated, a *justification* for the study is sometimes offered and a *review of the literature* can be included as a credit to the researcher for having some knowledge of what has been done in the past on this topic.

The *introduction* is dedicated to the history of the reseacher and his involvement with the topic. The *hypotheses* are those questions that were foremost in the mind of the researcher when he was uncovering the data. They are generally stated in concise expressions of FACTS about the variables of the investigation. Expressed *positively,* the researcher expects two variables to have *similarities*: Example: "There will be significant similarities between how males and females will vote on the bond issue."

Note that the term "will be" is used at the onset of the investigation. Later, the report will be stated in the past tense with the actual results. In the case stated above, the researcher *expected similarities* in the hypothesis stated. Had he *expected differences* in these results, he would have stated the same hypothesis thusly. Example: "There will be a significant difference between how males and females will vote on the bond issue."

The researcher can also set his own boundaries on what will be "significance." He may define less than 10 percent differences as significantly similar. And the differences greater than 10 percent as significantly different.

THE ORDER IN WHICH THE HYPOTHESES ARE STATED is important. That order is THEREAFTER the exact order in which all discussions take place. The hypotheses will set the procedure by which the data is gathered so as to determine differences and similarities between variables. The discussion format IS ALSO SET by the ordered sequence of the hypotheses.

So, too, are the review of the literature and the discussion of the results to follow the same ordered sequence as the hypotheses statements. They tell who will benefit directly from the information. They will also tell who could benefit indirectly from the information. This is sometimes the most important statement to make for researchers who wish to get financial support for the project. It cannot be assumed that everyone "knows" these things. "Everyone" does not. The best assumption is that "no one knows."

The *review of the literature* has it greatest advantage as being a credit to the researcher. It is an indication of his/her maturity, expertise, and competence. A good and well-written review helps to make the data more "believable."

2) *Procedure.* Discuss your instrument. Discuss what it is designed to probe. Discuss your design for gathering and treating the data. With relation to the treatment of the data, discuss the population or quality sampled. How was the population's representative sample selected? It is especially necessary to show that the representative sample was randomly selected.

3) *Results.* Discuss your results in everyday terms and plain language. Report the results as though you were telling it to a friend (placing in parentheses the exact results):

Examples:

A. Don't say, "Five out of sixteen females said yes to my first question while there were but nine of the nineteen males to answer yes to the question."

B. Do say, "Nearly a third (31%) of the females expressed the opinion that (say what the question revealed) while nearly half (47%) of the males were of the same opinion."

C. Percentages all have 100 as their common denominator. Taking the problem above:

Five of the sixteen: 500/16   = 31%
(If there were 100 females in this sample,
31 of them would have answered in this
manner).)

* * * * * *

Nine of the nineteen: 900/19   = 47%
(If there were 100 males in this sample,
47 of them would have answered in this
manner.)

D. The two sub-groups can now be compared in simple, obvious and clear language.

E. Display and illustrate these data with charts and/or graphs.

Normal, "J," and Bimodal (or "U") curves: What do they mean?

A normal curve (Figure 1A) distribution indicates the common occurrence of something being distributed with few individuals at either end and a rising number in the middle. A very peaked curve means fewer at either ends and more in the middle. A more gentle curve means more at either ends and fewer in the middle.

A bimodal or "U" curve (see Figure 1B), if thought of as upside-down normal curve, indicates just the opposite. In describing the diversity of a particular population, the largest numbers display the "different" characteristics while a few in the middle have mixed or hybrid characteristics.

Sometimes, depending on the way that the dichotomy or diversity is expressed, it could be displayed as either a normal curve or a "U" curve. If the data lends itself to this kind of choice, use the normal curve expression. People understand it better.

A "J" curve is an indication of little or no diversity. The population you are examining is mostly alike in the parameter it is displaying.

Conclusion. After you have mechanically discussed each hypothesis that was tested by your instruments (under Results, above), you may wish to express your own opinions concerning the trends among the different groups or subgroups

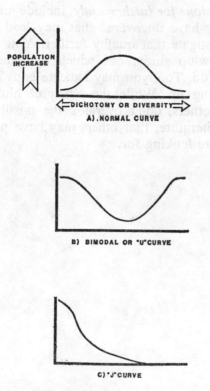

FIGURE 1

DISPLAYING THE DIVERSITIES OF A POPULATION

POPULATION
INCREASE

⇐DICHOTOMY OR DIVERSITY⇒

A). NORMAL CURVE

B) BIMODAL OR "U" CURVE

C) "J" CURVE

of data. These are YOUR CONCLUSIONS and may be written under that heading: "In the opinion of the writer . . ."

Discuss why you think that the results turned out the way that they did. HERE, FOR THE FIRST TIME IN YOUR PROJECT, and the only time, you are allowed your opinion. ELSEWHERE, YOU MUST NOT DEVIATE FROM WHAT THE DATA TELLS YOU TO SAY. Allow your data to speak for itself. It will tell you "what to say" and "how to say it."

The conclusion, like the introduction, is dedicated to the

researcher and his involvement with the project or topic. Yet another section could be included in the conclusion: *Suggestions for Further Study.*

In the *suggestions for further study,* include misconceptions your study may have uncovered that may lead one of your readers to investigate that quality further. You may wish to suggest a follow-up study, one which continues what you were unable to do. Too, you may indicate gaps in your study that need closing up. While these helpful hints are being passed on the others, don't overlook the possibilities, when reviewing the literature, that others may have passed on the "jewel" you were looking for.

Chapter 10

Science Projects: Compiling of Background Information (Compilation Research)

CONCEPTS

A. How to write a "paper" on a topic.
B. The activities involved in the writing of a paper resemble a review of literature phase of a scientific research or investigation project.
C. Take complete notes to avoid having to repeat activities.
D. How to cite sources.
E. Avoid plagiarizing someone else's work.

SKILLS AND PRINCIPLES

1. Using the reference books in gathering source materials.
2. Collecting ideas from source materials.
3. Citing the sources of materials from which came your ideas.
4. Citing sources and listing sources cited.
5. To copy someone else's work is to violate his copyright and this is breaking the law.

41

Comments for Students:

Another form of research that people do is just simply to write a "paper" on a topic. The expression means compiling a background of information and then formalizing it into a written report.

This project resembles the *review of literature* phase of a scientific research or investigation project. The only difference is that the person doing this kind of research, compilation research, may not intend to use the review for any other purpose than to learn something new about the topic. And, since he has it in his capacity to do so, he may wish to publish an article on the topic.

First thing to do is to decide on the topic. Next, start your review. Since the review of the literature is one of the major steps in this process, some pointers can be made about how to conduct these activities.

A good place to start is in *Readers' Guide, Biological and Agricultural Index,* or other reference books that the librarian can help you to locate. Be aware that few libraries have EVERY periodical (magazine) that will be mentioned as having an article on your topic. Know the limitations of your library. Then go after what is available.

When listing the articles that you find in a reference book, it usually pays to write down everything: author, the complete title of the article, name of the magazine, date, volume, and page number. It will keep you from having to go back and do it again later. The second or third time that this happens to you, you will begin to see the value of copying everything down when you can.

If you are keeping all of this information in a bound notebook, it will serve you well. If not, get a folder—one folder for each topic you are researching.

Once you have between six and a dozen articles listed—that number will depend on how much is written on your topic—start finding the various magazines and reading the articles. Reading can be done carefully or by scanning,

42

depending on the use you will make of the information contained.

Assuming that the information is important towards the completion of your compilation research project, start by taking down all of the vital information concerning the article. Example:

Author's Last Name, First Name and Middle Initial. "Title of the Article," *Name of the Journal,* Volume (Number): Inclusive Pages of the Article; Date of Journal.

Take notes below, listing in the margin the exact page from which each note is taken.

This procedure is necessary to save you a lot of time later. As you are writing your paper later, you will go from article to article, pulling out a sequence of ideas. The page number in the margin will be used when citing the exact source and page each idea comes from. Too, you have the inclusive pages for the bibliography (or sources cited) listing of each of your sources that you have used.

Be prepared to go into a scientific research project or investigation from such a project as this. Adjust the project to reflect the need for further study as evidence found in the literature merits it. Even if you were just going to write a paper, it is best that you design and gather data in support of your topic.

The format of a paper is similar to that of a research report in many ways. There should be the following suggested sections: introduction, review of the literature, text of report, and conclusions.

Cite All Sources. WHO says something is as important as WHAT is said. As you select ideas to include in your paper, it becomes increasingly important to identify the various sources of the blend of ideas.

Sometimes you will be given conflicting information in two or more of your sources. Which to use? If you have no other way of telling which is correct, you may accept the latest source as being "most probably the most accurate."

This will give you an idea why it is important to identify WHO your source is. Too, you may wish to report the conflicting information as you find it, citing the sources, and leaving it up to the reader to determine for himself how to use the information.

Citing Sources. There are several ways of citing sources, any of which is proper as long as all of the necessary information is given. It is recommended that a quick and easy way be used, if none other is called for specifically. If the information included in a citation is complete, it can easily be converted to any of the other methods OR STYLES of citing sources.

The use of footnotes at the bottom of a page or of endnotes at the end of the paper is likewise the author's choice. However, there are different ways of citing for different reasons and one becomes familiar with this aspect of writing with experience.

Plagiarizing. Throughout the world, copyrights protect authors from others taking and using their work without proper credit. Without going into the legal aspects of violating an individual's rights, the following discussion is simply made as an "awareness" statement.

A general rule of thumb is that you CANNOT COPY MORE THAN TEN CONSECUTIVE WORDS without being in violation of another person's copyrights. You may not use someone else's work and submit it in the guise of your own thoughts and words. You have inflicted an injury on another person. A law has been broken and you can be sued.

To copy someone's work and not to cite the source adds insult to injury. Use all of the ideas from wherever you can get them. However, be honest and give due credit to the author of each.

So far, everything emphasized was in the form of DON'Ts. You can communicate the same ideas and the same message.

44

However, it MUST BE in your words and not in the same words expressed in your sources.

You can paraphrase, or make parallel statements. You can also quote exactly what was said by someone else, as long as the author is fully credited for having written the idea.

Probably the most scholarly way to conduct these activities is to abstract your sources. Completely rewrite the ideas into your own expressions. Then use your sources to achieve your ends. Let them support you as examples one can find elsewhere, should he wish to read more about that specific topic.

If you enjoy writing, do it often. It probably doesn't come that naturally for anyone. However, with practice comes professional growth in your own way and your own style. No two writers are the same because of our individual differences.

Chapter 11

Science Fair Projects: Displaying a Scientific Concept

CONCEPTS

A. A good project does not come from out of the blue —review the literature.
B. Approach the project with phases: review literature, construct a research design, gather data, process the data, construct a display model, build the real model.
C. Facts about the "displayed" science fair project.

SKILLS AND PRINCIPLES

1. Select the MAJOR or BIG IDEA of the project.
2. Make a simple statement of this idea.
3. Build the project display around this idea.
4. Once it is known WHAT to display, consider TO WHOM and start with sketches, proceed to blueprints, and then to a model.
5. Balance the display objects using colors, tones and textures.
6. The kinds of questions asked by viewers tell much about the successes and failures in communicating the ideas. RECORD THESE QUESTIONS.

7. Immediately after this year's event, start planning for next year.

Comments for Students:

All of the previous chapters were intended to be understood prior to reading this one. They help you with selecting, preparing and executing a project. The execution of a project gives you data. Other chapters give you pointers on processing the data and writing them up in the form of a report.

If you have done all or at least most of these things, you are now ready to consider displaying your project. The one thing that has been emphasized the most up to this point has been THE DATA. Now, you will wish to use the data to develop a conceptual message—an idea. What was the biggest idea of your findings? It is around this big idea that you will build your science fair project.

In essence, consider this. YOU SHOULD DISPLAY YOUR PROJECT TO INCLUDE THE RESULTS AND FINDINGS IN SUCH A MANNER THAT A VIEWER CAN UNDERSTAND THEM IN FIVE TO TEN SECONDS. He should be able to walk away at that time and be informed about: 1) what you did, 2) how you did it, and 3) what your results were.

Different displays differ for different reasons. You may have a number of reasons for building a display. However, in most cases a display is a display and approach is the same, or similar, with little regard as to why. One of the few differences from display to display would be the audience for whom it is designed.

How to Display Your Idea. It is assumed that you know WHAT you will be displaying and TO WHOM or FOR WHOM it is designed to reach. It is also assumed that you will want to get a message across. That is the WHAT, above.

Start with a sketch of your early ideas. Include pictures, written messages, labels, and write in a title. Decide on how

47

to sequence your viewer's attention—from left to right and top to bottom are "normal" for our society.

Displaying your project will draw on your knowledge of art: colors, tones, and textures. Physically balance all of your display items that they neatly occupy a balance in positions— not too heavy on one or the other side and evenly distributed.

Try the display on a friend. On your teacher(s)—especially an art teacher if possible. Check out the validity of the statements you make. And the spelling!

Does your display INTRODUCE a new topic? Does it bring new interest to a well-known topic? Does it display the skills needed to master the topic? Does it reach the desired audience? It is too cluttered or too sparsely scattered?

Build a cardboard model or a blueprint diagram of each refined version. Always keep in mind the five to ten second rule. That's about all of the time you will get from MOST of your viewers.

Building good science fair projects takes more than one year of experience. So, be aware that some of the questions that viewers will ask you are clues for improvement.

If you are asked about the procedure in obtaining data, it means that you failed to communicate this fact of your project. Keep a record of all the questions that are asked. They tell you two things—either you failed to communicate in different ways or you did communicate and the viewers understood your project well. Review your questions at the end of this fair and immediately start on next year's project.

Part II

Teacher's Materials Advance Concepts: Dichotomies in Education; Plenty of Room for Everyone

Part II

Teacher's Material Advance Concepts: Dichotomies in Education; Plenty of Room for Everyone

Chapter 12

Teaching-Learning Modes As Applied in a Teaching-Learning Environment

When one is defining a philosophy of education, either "the teaching act" or "the learning act" takes priority in that expression. For the educator where the teaching strategy and classroom activities are teacher-dominated, teacher-oriented, or teacher-structured, the teaching act will include the learning act by definition. A topic covered presumes a topic learned by all students (or at least the ones that count—the bright ones).

For the educator where the teaching strategy and classroom activities are student-oriented or student-structured, the learning act takes priority when defining education. In this classroom, student ideas and input take an active part in the curriculum.

Teaching Modes:

Three classroom modes are suggested which are closely oriented to the familiar conservative, electric, and liberal philosophies (see Figure 2). These educational modes, or philosophies, are herein referred to, respectively, as "authoritarian, eclectic, and self-directed."

51

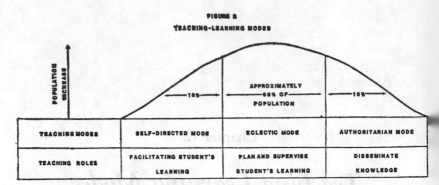

FIGURE 2
TEACHING-LEARNING MODES

These three philosophies (actually two extremes with a hybrid center) exist with all shades of possibilities in between. An individual teacher performs actively within a definite range on the continuum base between the two extremes (after Sonnier, 1975, p. 221; see also Davies, p. 177).

The *authoritarian and self-directed modes* give at least an appearance of being diverging or opposite end-poles of the same phenomena. They will be described first. Since the *eclectic mode* appears to be the intermeshing middle, it will be described last.

The *authoritarian mode* represents the classroom in which the teacher's role is to disseminate facts and knowledge. This occurs in the teacher-centered classroom in which cognitive domain objectives dominate the content to be learned.

The *self-directed mode* has the entire focus of learning in the hands of the learner, himself. The teacher's role is to facilitate the student's learning with affective domain objectives dominating over cognitive domain objectives. A pattern often emerges of: 1) planning; 2) searching, collecting, and compiling; and 3) sharing these findings with other students. At its best, this pattern is initiated over and over again by groups as well as by individuals. The self-directed teacher sees himself as a facilitator of the student's learning.

The *eclectic mode* represents a classroom in which the teacher's role is to supervise the student's learning. This could be done in either a teacher-centered or a student-and-teacher-centered classroom. An eclectic teacher can function comfortably within that implied range somewhere between the two extremes, authoritarian and self-directed. The majority of the teachers (68 percent —see Figure 2) practice this mode. Another way to describe the eclectic philosophy of education is by the adage "the best of the old and the good of the new."

Range of Operation and Philosophical Position:

These three philosophies (herein suggested to be two extremes with a hybrid center) exist with all shades of position in between. An individual teacher performs activities within a definite range on a continuum base between these two extremes. This is to be considered as that teacher's *range of operation*. With the range of operation established, the center of this range is his *philosophical position*. One's philosophical position could be located anywhere on the continuum.

The range of operation varies greatly from teacher to teacher. Even though one's range of operation could span two philosophies, the philosophical position can almost always be identified with one or the other of the three philosophies. Generally speaking, most teachers are eclectic and sufficiently flexible to function in more than one mode. However, they are more oriented or committed to one mode than to the other.

Teaching Modes and Learning Theories:

When reviewing and interpreting the learning theories, problems arise. If one considers "how human beings learn," neither the self-directed nor the authoritarian mode can be justified. This does not take away from the "few" capable teachers who have high levels of achievement in these modes. It is proposed, however, that many teachers practice at these extremes without the necessary philosophy and talent.

Teachers with a high level of achievement in the authoritarian mode who have good rapport with students should be encouraged to continue to practice in this mode. Most of these teachers, however, should turn to the eclectic mode for an even greater degree of success with students and a greater

53

psychological and philosophical satisfaction. The same analogy can be made concerning the self-directed mode, sometimes called "Laissez-Faire."

Teaching Mode and Lesson Plan Objectives:

Teachers who prefer to structure the learning experiences of students should be aware of the types of objectives which they write or imply in their lesson plans. The lesson plans which best suit the philosophical and psychological needs of this teacher are with cognitive objectives that are "task" or "performance oriented." Since this teacher does not turn to the student for the curriculum content or mode of instruction, it would not be in keeping to place a major emphasis on objectives that are "affective" or designed to develop "attitude."

There is a small segment of the teaching population that is practicing in the authoritarian mode—those with conviction. There are many others practicing in that mode, but only in transition from one educational movement to another—mostly eclectic individuals.

The authoritarian mode has its deepest roots in contemporary activities such as programmed and computer-assisted learning, educational television, the writing of performance objectives, competency-based teaching, and accountability.

Since, in the self-directed mode the teacher's role is to facilitate learning, it should be obvious that this is a student-centered classroom. The student's objective, often affective and attitude developing, plays a major role in the content of the course. This mode is also represented by a small segment of the teaching profession.

SKILLS AND PRINCIPLES

1. Distinguish between the teaching act and the learning act when dispensing knowledge in the educational enterprise.
2. Distinguish between a student-oriented learning environment and a teacher-centered learning environment.
3. Distinguish between authoritarian, eclectic and self-directed learning environment and teaching environment.

54

Chapter 13

Logic Patterns and Individual Differences

Individual differences may be due to differences in logic patterns which are proposed to be genetically based. Two extreme, mutually exclusive, pure form of thought patterns are proposed for consideration.

In this model, most individuals display intermediate traits of these two qualities, "creative and constructive" (see Figure 2). An understanding of these qualities could add to the success of both educator and student. This understanding would further provide meaning to the concept that individuals learn differently and that their instructional processes and format needs are likewise different.

Traditionally, educational practices have displayed varying forms of group instruction based on the assumption that all students, under a given experience, learn in the same way and/or at the same time. The educational experience rendered to (or for) the learner was planned in advance so as to maintain some degree of control over the learning activity according to a definite, ordered pattern.

These practices continue to be the universal teaching strategy. A logical pattern of thought such as the following would summarize the prevailing instructional philosophy

55

(Figure3): If A = B and B = C, these being facts with a concept, then A = C, the concept or the big idea.

There is exhibited little or no concern for the possibility that all students do not think by the foregoing logic pattern. It is proposed that there exist different logic patterns among different individuals. It is in everyone to possess wisdom—different wisdoms and by different degrees. As applied to education, consideration of these differences could give meaning to the concept that individuals learn differently and that their instructional process and format needs differ.

There have been many reports of divergent needs on the part of both the teacher and students. Meeting these needs is still in the realm of opinion. There exists a paradox in that proponents of the open system of education must tolerate highly structured operations whereas proponents of the highly structured system cannot tolerate openness (see Chapter 15 for more on "open education").

A Paradigm Based on the Syllogism. The prevailing instructional philosophy is one that coincides with the syllogism (If A = B and B = C, then, A = C). The possibility is raised that some individuals instantly see that A = C without the minutia involved in A = B and B = C, and they are bored by the details. If allowed to proceed with a problem or an investigation, on their own, they will come to the conclusion: therefore, A = B and B = C. This is related to the well-known inductive-deductive concept of reality.

In the flexibility of an individual's mind, creativity requires a visualizing or synthesizing (inductive) ability while the counterpart of creativity, constructivity, requires an analyzing (deductive) ability. Creativity is a diverging process and constructivity is a covering process (see Chapter 14).

It is proposed that the deductive thought process, as expressed in the syllogism, is the common reasoning process in individuals that are extremely methodical as in the finest tradition of mathematics, accounting, engineering, and physics, just to mention a few personal persuasions. These individuals do well in the existing educational format and

56

FIGURE 3
A MODEL OF DIFFERENT LOGIC
PATTERNS IN DIVERGENT INDIVIDUALS

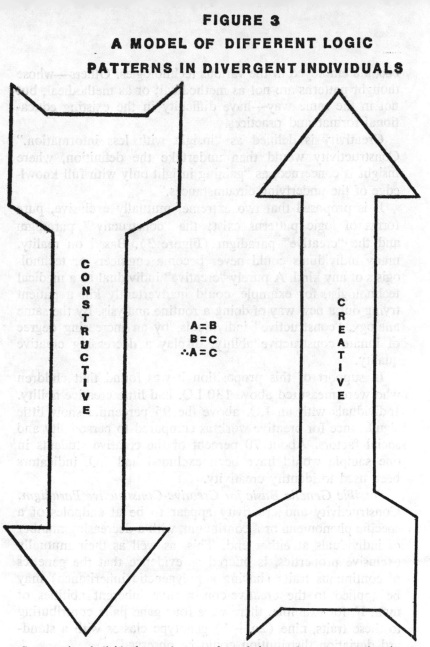

$$A = B$$
$$B = C$$
$$\therefore A = C$$

Constructive individuals need more factual input than do creative individuals in determining or constructing a concept. This is a converging or deductive process. Creative individuals can determine or construct a concept with less mental input or information. This is a diverging or inductive process. Too, the modes of conceptual realization may likewise differ (after Sonnier, 1976, p. 139).

FIGURE 3

become employed in the various technologies. Others—whose thought patterns are not as methodical; or as methodical, but not in the same way—have difficulty in the existing educational format and practices.

Creativity is defined as "insight with less information." Constructivity would then undertake the definition, where insight is concerned, as "gaining insight only with full knowledge of the underlying circumstances."

It is proposed that two extreme, mutually exclusive, pure forms of logic patterns exist: the "constructive" paradigm and the "creative" paradigm (Figure 3). Based on reality, many individuals could never become engineers or technologists of any kind. A purely "creative" individual as a medical technologist, for example, could inadvertently kill a patient trying out a new way of doing a routine analysis. By the same analogy, "constructive" individuals, by an increasing degree of innate constructive ability, display a decreasing creative quality.

In support of this proposition it was found that children who were measured above 130 I.Q. had little creative ability. Individuals with an I.Q. above the 95 percentile show little significance for creative work as compared to personality and social factors. About 70 percent of the creative students in one sample would have been excluded had I.Q. indicators been used to identify creativity.

Possible Genetic Basic for Creative-Constructive Paradigm. Constructivity and creativity appear to be at endpoles of a specific phenomena or a continuum, with a decreasing number of individuals at either end. This, as well as their mutually exclusive properties, is offered as evidence that the genetics of continuous traits (having a polygenetic inheritance) may be applied to the creative-constructive inherent abilities of man. If, for example, there were four gene pairs contributing to these traits, nine $(2n + 1)$ genotype classes with a standard deviation distribution could be observed.

If there were three gene pairs, seven $(2n = 1)$ genotypes could be observed (see Figure 4). However, both the truth

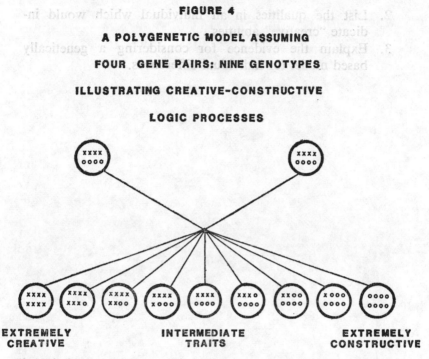

FIGURE 4

A POLYGENETIC MODEL ASSUMING

FOUR GENE PAIRS: NINE GENOTYPES

ILLUSTRATING CREATIVE-CONSTRUCTIVE

LOGIC PROCESSES

EXTREMELY CREATIVE

INTERMEDIATE TRAITS

EXTREMELY CONSTRUCTIVE

If the logic process were to be a continuous or polygenetic heredity and there were (for example only) four gene pairs involved, nine genotype classes would result with the two phenotype traits at either end and all other possessing intermediate traits of the creative-constructive quality (after Sonnier, 1976, p. 141).

of the matter and the number of gene pairs are yet in need of demonstration.

A good way to view the fixed intelligence question is by analogy with a hand of cards. "Heredity deals the cards and the environment plays with them." A good hand can be abused and meet with misfortune while a poor hand can meet with nothing but success—pointing to extreme cases.

SKILLS AND PRINCIPLES

1. List the qualities in an individual which would indicative "creative" abilities.

2. List the qualities in an individual which would indicate "creative" abilities .
3. Explain the evidence for considering a genetically
   based model for individual differences.

Chapter 14

The Creative-Constructive Model: As Applied in a Teaching-Learning Environment

Assuming that most individuals display a blend of the creative and constructive traits and that there are a few individuals at either end of the continuum with a high innate ability in one of the traits, a partial list of contributing factors of each trait can be catalogued, as well as the assumed rate of occurrence by standard deviation (see Figure 5).

It is proposed that most individuals display intermediate traits of the creative-constructive paradigm. However, the possibility is left open for the existence of other basic logic patterns among mankind.

The Constructive paradigm. Constructive individuals build upon the existing mental structures with little or no capacity for deviation. They perform well in a wide range of tasks from routine to highly skilled levels of technology such as engineering. They build bridges and buildings well, as if with programmed knowledge. However, the construction of a "new kind" of building presents obscure and abstract conceptions for these individuals.

In the context of Figure 5, they indicate a preference for mental processes that are deductive in nature, analyzing and

61

FIGURE 5

A CREATIVE-CONSTRUCTIVE MODEL OF HUMAN BEHAVIOR

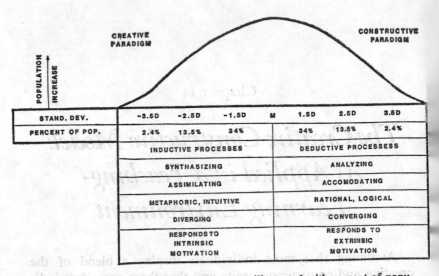

STAND. DEV.	-3.5D	-2.5D	-1.5D	M	1.5D	2.5D	3.5D
PERCENT OF POP.	2.4%	13.5%	34%		34%	13.5%	2.4%
	INDUCTIVE PROCESSES				DEDUCTIVE PROCESSESS		
	SYNTHASIZING				ANALYZING		
	ASSIMILATING				ACCOMODATING		
	METAPHORIC, INTUITIVE				RATIONAL, LOGICAL		
	DIVERGING				CONVERGING		
	RESPONDS TO INTRINSIC MOTIVATION				RESPONDS TO EXTRINSIC MOTIVATION		

The creative and constructive paradigms are illustrated with percent of population per standard deviation in a normally distributed population (after Sonnier, 1976, p. 142).

accommodating. They prefer doing activities that are rational and logical and activities that require converging thinking.

As a student, such an individual would respond more attentively to teachers that make education extrinsically motivating (challenging). This individual finds "problem solving" a rewarding activity.

Concerning social structuredness, if forced into action through confrontation, the radical of this group would turn to standard and proven structures (tradition) for the solution of problems—an activity that herein defines the constructive paradigm.

The Creative Paradigm. The mathematical application of physical reality is not out of reach for the creative individual. However, the highly rational and logical tasks on which constructive individuals thrive are obscure and abstract conceptions for this individual. Too, he has as little capacity for deviation as does a constructive individual.

The creative individual would have to be intrinsically motivated or "turned on" to a specific discipline before spending any time studying it. He could, for example, study muscles of the human body if such a study were to enable him to draw or paint a better figure of a man. He would study physics of light or gravity if such a study were to meet a specific intrinsic need.

Creative individuals indicate a greater need to retain their individuality. This is a primary source of conflict with constructive individuals, who like the organizaton and personal surrender of military life, civic groups and activities as well as political gatherings.

The preferred mental processes for the creative individual are metaphoric, intuitive, inductive, synthesizing, assimilating, and doing activities that require diverging through processes.

Creative individuals respond positively to teaching modes that accommodate their need to be intrinsically motivated. Upon confrontation, radicals of this innate persuasion tend to tear down the established social and educational format with what is to them a perfect vision or insight of what the new ones are to be like—this is creativity by definition.

Implication for Education. Taking into consideration environmental factors, some individuals have a greater range to develop innate creative-constructive traits than do others. The population curve is probably shifted to the conservative, or constructive, side in that education is an institution that must perpetuate itself.

This may mean that there are some creative individuals operating in the constructive paradigm, a philosophical contradiction that seeds psychological difficulties. Should this be the case, it may shed light on at least some of the institution's "rough edges."

Many criticisms have been leveled at our preoccupation with an institution that operated in the dominantly constructive paradigm. While it may have contributed significantly

63

to human progress, as we know it to date, it may have also inadvertently maintained conditions that inhibit self-evaluation and the fulfillment of innate individual potentials.

As concerned with individual differences, educational processes and needs differ. There is an emerging conflict of interest concerning the desirable degree of classroom structure. This also appears to be a two-ended phenomena: teacher-structure vs. student-structure. With the application of the creative-construction paradigm, education is at its very best for the constructive teacher when it is highly structured. Individual differences are met through a sensitive awareness of as many of the students as possible in a concerted effort to achieve the teacher's expected goals in the cognitive domain.

For the creative teacher, the degree of structuredness has its origin in the students themselves. Individual differences are met through the student's personal involvement in the affective domain. Individual or group-derived goals may or may not be in concert with the rest of the class. For the eclectic teacher, these distinctions are of little concern.

Indications are that a teacher must practice in a philosophical mode commensurate with his innate logic pattern: authoritarian, eclectic, or self-directed (see Figure 2). By so doing, however, he may inadvertently impose upon his students the task of having philosophical and psychological compatibility with himself. However, this does not create a problem for students of different persuasions, as long as the teacher is practicing firmly within the paradigm for which he is best suited and if there is an atmosphere of mutual respect.

Personality problems arise when a teacher is practicing a different philosophy or paradigm. If a difficulty arises, they (teacher and students) could be forced into confrontation with the students being in captive attendance. It may be inserted here that a person with a "bad attitude" is usually a person with a different set of values.

It is in this atmosphere of misunderstanding that brigand students are created and that discipline problems are nurtured.

64

Untold damage may have resulted from discrimination because of this lack of the knowledge of how to develop the different innate abilities of different individuals.

The purpose of these discussions is not to adversely criticize the various forms of institutional structures, but to lend meaning and purpose to their existence in the light of distinct innate human differences. By understanding the foregoing paradigms, teachers may avoid personal conflicts that may lead to confrontations with students and colleagues.

It is the student for whom we must show our highest concern.

Both the creative and the constructive student are in our classroom at all levels of education. And, most individuals, teachers and students, innately behave with patterns from one or another of these paradigms. This is "society's healthy blend." It was upon this precise concept that our educational institutions were founded—for the fulfillment of each, according to his potentials.

The right of each student to develop his own innate potential must no longer be denied. Individuals with extreme creative or constructive traits tend to be "different" and misunderstood. The confusion and difficulty that are created for some individuals by our educational institutions may not be necessary.

Birth control, euthanasia, women's rights, the inequality of wealth, as well as some of the other institutional problems that involve the person will continue to plague our society until all individual differences are accepted as "society's healthy blend." It has been repeatedly demonstrated that human differences have a way of being magnified by confrontation—and literally eliminated by understanding.

With respect to individual differences, it has been said that there is work to be done in education and that it will be the reformers (eclectic), not the reactionaries (authoritarian) or the revolutionaries (self-directed), who will accomplish it. It was implied further that without the revolutionary there would be no change. Without the reactionary, the change would be meaningless.

SKILLS AND PRINCIPLES

1. List the preference-activities of the constructive paradigm.
2. List the preference-activities of the creative paradigm.
3. List the preference-activities for teachers who prefer a teacher-structured classroom setting.
4. List the preference-activities for teachers who prefer a student-structured classroom setting.
5. List how the eclectic teacher fits in these patterns of preference-activities.
6. List the justifications for providing and allowing this wide range of teacher-preferences in classroom environments.

Chapter 15

Why Open Education

The term "open" has meant different things to different people—each person thinking of himself as being an "open" person. Therefore, it has almost as many meanings as persons referring to their own quality and quantity "openness."

The authoritarian is not inclined to "opening" his content to the scrutiny of students. It is not in his nature to do so, which is understood by both teacher and student. He has, however, other means of opening education. He does this by way of the physical environment—"open space."

In this sense, open education means movable walls and a mobile classroom—here, there, or anywhere. This mobility includes the great outdoors as a teaching-learning environment. However, course content and teaching strategy retain their stability. This is one of the ways that the authoritarian teacher has of including affective objectives in his lesson plans.

The self-directed person points to the head when he means "open." Openness means the freedom to expand at the will of the individual, making reference to curricular alternatives on the individual's level. These efforts, in a nutshell, emphasize two qualities: personal growth and sharing knowledge with others.

The eclectic person can live with the self-directed point of view, to some extent. To him, however, the concept takes the shape of "open-ended investigation" with "discovery" being at the end of the tunnel. The structure could well be "locked-

67

step," with the entire group achieving a common teacher-directed goal.

The quality and quantity of openness herein recommended calls for open-mindedness to individual differences. However, group structure could take whatever direction that the instructor terms desirable.

It is worthy of note that there is one common thread of opinion among educators of these diverse philosophies. *Openness is almost always related with group activities.* This places a great importance on and points to the value of *group interaction* in the classroom.

Therefore, it is strongly recommended that each teacher use student groups in achieving at least some of their educational goals. Since this is a commonly used practice, with different ways and different reasons for different teachers, its values are almost universally *accepted.*

There is something motivating about students working and sharing with students. And there is excitement in any teacher seeing motivated students. However, these lofty plans and activities depend heavily on the skills of the teacher for organizing and maintaining momentum.

Teachers of all philosophical diversities group students in learning activities from time to time. The purposes, goals, and end products may vary. But grouping in teaching-learning environments occurs in nearly all classrooms, some more than others, with the frequency related to the managerial skills of the teacher. In general, these are the "issues" of "open" education.

It is extremely desirable that each teacher practice and improve group managerial skills. The earlier chapters of this textbook have provided a number of experiences that lead toward the achievement of this goal.

SKILLS AND PRINCIPLES

1. Identify the dichotomies of "open" education.
2. Identify the modes of opening educational opportunities.
3. List some of the ways that you could improve upon your group managerial skills.

Chapter 16

The Nature of Human Brain Hemispheres: The Basis for Some Individual Differences

The human brain is divided into two distinct hemispheric sections that are physically connected with each other by a a large bundle of nerve fibers called the *corpus callosum*. Although this physical connection would appear to be significant in the thought processes, little is known concerning the interactions of the two hemispheres by way of the corpus callosum.

Each hemisphere is the seat of a large number of operations in the thought processes and body functions. However, they are different with each side having its own set of complex controls—one side knowing what the other is doing largely subconsciously.

There were three stages of development in the discovery of brain lateralization or hemisphericity—to express two of the commonly used terms. Clinical psychologists had l o n g suspected the dual nature of human consciousness. Early in their studies, the left and right hemispheres were dubbed the "major" and "minor" hemispheres, respectively.

A second discovery whittled the knowledge more keenly. The two hemispheres were found to be "equal," which dispelled the major-minor misnomer, although slowly. The work of neurologists and neurosurgeons revealed that when the left cerebral hemisphere was damaged, to some degree—slightly to totally, language and mathematical abilities were hampered.

Damage to the right cerebral hemisphere consistantly interfered with visual-spatial mentation—color, shapes, identifying faces, and such tasks as dressing oneself adequately. Persons with such damage retained unimpaired speech and reasoning abilities.

A third stage of information came from unilateral shock treatments that temporarily "freeze" one side or the other in order to continue the kind of investigations that had been started by neurosurgeons. As a result of all this information the educational implications of this knowledge continue to be developed and refined by many individuals and research groups.

What we know, basically, is that the left brain hemisphere characteristically

is the center for language and speech;
controls logical, linear, analytical, and sequential thinking;
controls the right side of the body.

The right hemisphere characteristically

controls orientation in space;
recognizes faces, shapes, colors, textures, and musical pitch;
controls many of our emotions;
controls the left side of our body;
emits holistic thought (visualizes the thought).

While each one of us has one or the other of our hemispheres as "the dominant one," the world places different emphases on the importance of the hemispheric characteristics in education, philosophy and social interactions of people. These are environmental pressures imposed onto our innate being.

In the Western culture, namely Europe and the Americas, a great deal of emphasis is placed on the left hemispheric functions. Considering that the left brain controls the right side of the body, is it any wonder that a military salute is rendered with the right hand, or that we are a "right-handed" society?

Conversely, Asians place much of this kind of emphasis on holistic thinking. Arts and crafts, visualizing abilities, and other "right brain" characteristics dominate family and educational priorities, in general.

There is evidence that the Japanese and Polynesian languages have common ancestories in that they are both vowel sounding and are purposefully pronounced with natural sounds such as those of crickets, birds, ocean waves, and others. Thus, vowels, consonants, animal s o u n d s, and Japanese and Polynesian music are all processed in the left hemisphere. In Japanese and Polynesian societies, children learn their language during the formal education years by listening and speaking it. Other Asians and Westerners learn by reading and writing it.

For these reasons, it has been determined that the Japanese and Polynesians process all of these sounds in their left hemisphere because of their communicative and/or language nature. With this interpretation, it should come as little or no surprise that they also process mechanical sounds—e.g., bells, whistles, and helicopter noises—in their right hemisphere as do other world ethnic groups.

We know that children come into the world with a "clear slate," so far as symbols are concerned. Language and mathematical skills must be developed later. The child is totally dependent on the right hemisphere which seems to be readily available.

As the left brain develops with speech, reading, writing, and mathematics skills, so does holistic or visualizing thought —with each experience. We know that girls mature faster into this transition than boys—but that boys, by junior high school age, catch up and do as well.

We are also learning that a few persons, corresponding to the minorities at either end of the creative-constructive model of human behaviour (see Figure 5), have two right brains and are extremely visual in personal characteristics.

It was found that children, under these conditions, learn to

71

read late and may be labeled "dyslexic." After a few bouts in "special education" classes, these children sometimes end up doing as well as others. By late junior high school age they can no longer be distinguished as being "academically different."

Too, there are some, a small number of individuals, born with two left hemispheres. At early childhood, these individuals, go after symbols with a ferocious appetite. Some even teach themselves to read, having available visual aids like childrens' books in the environment.

A number of attempts have been made to identify "brain dominance" in individuals. There would seem to be an "obvious" relationship with either being right- or left-handed.

This is not so. A number of problems arise, the first being an unsympathetic mother with a left-handed baby. The few that survive this ordeal have other reasons for being left-handed; and would individuals with two right or two left hemispheres display mixed dominance or non-dominance?

It has been determined that human beings are born "normally" with the left hemisphere as their analyzing side and the right as their visualizing side. Note the term "normally." Conceivably, there are individuals normal in every way, except that their right hemisphere is their analyzing side and their left is their visualizing side.

Consider one of these individuals with a dominant analyzing hemisphere on the right side. If allowed to be so by his mother, he will be left-handed. Most anlyzing individuals are right-handed.

The vast number of individuals (the peak of the population curve in Figure 5) are with m i x e d dominant hemispheric characteristics. One of these individuals could aim a gun with the left eye, kick a ball with the right foot, and be left-handed.

Mixed dominance also explains ambidextrous individuals. However, one should not overlook the fact that some individuals "train" themselves that way. By training, they are more effectively ambidextrous than others that were born with greater innate potentials.

Typing and piano playing are examples of tasks requiring

a high degree of right-left side training. It would make sense that learning how to type or to play the piano would come easier for individuals who have mixed dominance.

However, individual determination probably plays as great a role as innate ability. Perhaps, it may be said of all of these skills, as with other "lateralization" traits, "heredity deals the cards and the environment plays them."

Too, the academic question is raised: What are the resulting consequences on personality development of physically handicapped individuals? How does myopic vision or astigmatism affect the personality development of an extremely visually oriented individual? This opens an entirely new way of looking at these problems.

SKILLS AND PRINCIPLES

1. Describe the physical appearance of the two brain hemispheres and its apparent significance in brain lateralization, or hemisphericity, with relations to the thought processes.
2. Describe the stages of development of our knowledge of lateralization.
3. List the characteristics of the left brain hemisphere.
4. List the cultural manifestations of importance of these characteristics.
5. How may some individuals of our culture be affected by these value judgements of importance?
6. How could dominance of one hemisphere over the other contribute to individual differences?

73

Chapter 17

Teach the Left Brain and Only the Left Brain Learns — Teach the Right Brain and Both Brains Learn

It is all but established that the left brain hemisphere of humans processes verbal-sequential data and that the discretely different right brain processes visual-spatial data. And, there is evidence that we use one hemisphere more effectively than the other as a factor of individual differences. In other words, some individuals have a dominant right hemisphere and are visually oriented, while others have a dominant left hemisphere and are more verbally oriented and are perhaps more innately literary.

There is a great deal of confusion today concerning the education of children. Researchers in science education agree that many students *are not* being reached. There is, however, little agreement as to why this is true or what should be done to eliminate the problem.

Research concerning the hemisphericity of the human brain has provided some insight into possible explanations for the reason why many children are not succeeding in today's schools. It was theorized that teachers are using mostly left hemisphere input and output in their instructional strategies—the cognitive domain.

This is handicapping all learners because nearly every child has at least some capacity to learn to use his hight hemisphere. However, many learners are particularly handicapped because they learn best through right hemisphere input—the affective domain.

The term "listening-learners" suits well these individuals. Their listening abilities are so acute that they "see the world" through their ears. Unless this is understood by EVERY EARLY CHILDHOOD TEACHER, the children (and the institution) will have problems.

Simply stated, teaching strategies that employ objectives of the cognitive domain mostly affect the left hemisphere. However, teaching strategies that employ objectives of the affective domain affect both, the right and the left hemisphere. The latter implies the use of any number of tactics such as the humanistic approach; hands-on; learn by doing; or, the all encompassing term, holistic education.

There is growing concern that since 1969 there hase been a decline in the science knowledge of students aged 9 through 17 years based on the results of a survey by the National Assessment of Educational Progress. Other surveys indicate that a majority of the non-science majors in college have a negative attitude toward science and are hesitant to enroll in science courses.

This noninterest might be explained by the inadequacies of the teaching strategies that are generally used in teaching science. The usual approach is logical, linear, and numerical in nature (the cognitive domain) and ignores the use of the imagination, visualization, and sensory abilities of students (the affective domain).

In order for the capabilties of all students to be developed, teaching strategies must be designed and curriculum materials developed to involve both hemispheres of the brain in the learning process. The best method of instruction should integrate the functions of the two brain hemispheres in a bal-

75

FIGURE 6

A POLYGENETIC MODEL ASSUMING

FOUR GENE PAIRS: NINE GENOTYPES

ILLUSTRATING HEMISPHERIC DOMINANCES

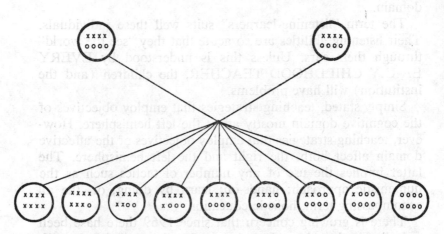

If hemispheric dominance were to be a continuous or polygenetic heredity and there were (for example only) four gene pairs involved, nine genotype classes would result with the two phenotype traits at either end, all others would possess intermediate traits of the visual-spatial and verbal-sequential qualities (marginal to non-dominance).

anced manner, apparently achieved through the affective domain.

Human children may be born right-hemisphere oriented. Evidence for this includes the fact that in 80 percent of the cases newborn infants tend to position t h e i r left ear up in order to channel sounds input into their right b r a i n hemisphere. The first forms of communication for children are nonverbal and involve the right hemisphere. These traits may well be genetically based (see Figure 6).

When children enter school they are encouraged to drop their sensory-imaginative talents and develop verbal-numerical skills. The effects of the hemisphericity of the brain seems to increase with age in children. The greatest difference has been noted between the fourth and sixth grades.

The shift from right hemisphere orientation to the left is difficult for many students. Furthermore, some students are right-hemisphere dominant and are unable to make the shift effectively. Consequently, they are discriminated against by today's school standards. There is also evidence that the urban poor tend to be right-hemisphere oriented, while middle-class individuals are more left-hemisphere oriented, *an indication of environmental factors.*

There is also evidence for sexual differences in the development of hemispheric dominance. Boys show right dominance (visual-spatial processing) while girls show bilateral representation until thirteen. While this explains what we already know about individual and sex differences, provisions are yet to be made for these needs in today's schools.

Dyslexic children (children with special reading problems) appear to have two "right" brain hemispheres. As can be expected, these children are strongly visual-spatial oriented and are listening-learners. Yet, they grow into the teen ages as "normal" individuals. However, the lost years may take their toll among many of these children.

If these indications and assumptions are true, it would thus be discriminatory to insist that all children must adapt to a left hemisphere mode of instruction and learning. *There is evidence that data input of the right hemisphere may readily stimulate both hemispheres while it may be more difficult for left hemisphere input data to stimulate the right hemisphere.* Assuming that this is true, there is yet another way to interpret these data. Simply expressed: "Teach the left brain and only the left brain learns—teach the right brain and both brains learn."

This aphorism would be true only for the vast majority of persons with neither right nor left hemisphere dominance. Persons at either extreme of this model would possess characteristics of extreme visual-spatial and verbal-sequential rationality. However, they too can be educated in a classroom at-

77

mosphere with a teaching strategy that is sensitive to the education of both hemispheres—strategies employing objectives in the affective domain.

The polygenetic model assuming four gene pairs in explaining individual differences in logic paterns could apply to hemisphericity as well. That model would also explain the increasing number of individuals with intermediate traits of visual-spatial and verbal-sequential and the decreasing number of individuals with either one of these mutually exclusive traits (see Figures 4 and 6).

SKILLS AND PRINCIPLES

1. Describe the nature of the left brain hemisphere.
2. Describe the nature of the right brain hemisphere.
3. Describe the behaviour of a student who has a dominant right hemisphere.
4. Describe the behaviour of a student who has a dominant right hemisphere.
5. How can lower elementary teachers best serve the listening-learners' limitations?

Chapter 18

Analyzers and Visualizers

The concluding statement about educating both brains is that there are basically two mutually exclusive and conflicting factors contributing toward individual differences. Some persons are MOST OF THE TIME analyzers. Others are MOST OF THE TIME visualizers.

The most probable cause for these qualities being so elusive to educational research is that analyzers can also visualize and visualizers can also analyze. This point is an ever-present obstacle in explaining the split-brain theory as it applies to education. It is this parameter which muddies the waters and hampers the complete acceptance and credibility of educating both brains.

Too, this is precisely why we should teach both brains, with full understanding of the split-brain theory and do it with vigor. Indeed, it is MOST DESIRABLE for persons to be agile analyzers and at the same time visualizers, and vice versa.

However, our society places its complete thrust in an educational institution which nurtures and fosters analyzing as THE ONLY real and basic value. Visualizing does not even approach a second place in educational objectives.

As hard as some teachers try to educate the "whole child," the end product is almost evidently that the analyzing hemisphere gets all of the attention. While this is done at the expense of educating both brains, it need not be so.

79

The most important point to be made is that both brains can be educated to function effectively for the welfare of each and everyone of us. We could all prosper from an educational institutional which sharpens one's ability to analyze while at the same time mustering one's abilities towards being a better visualizer.

As applied to what we already know about educating both brains, this means that if we teach persons to analyze—i.e., teaching the left brain—the only product of this effort is more effective powers in analyzing. Naturally, there can be little criticism of this effort nor of the educational product. However, this is NOT ENOUGH.

Here's the real message. If we teach persons to visualize, their analyzing powers are simultaneously fostered! "Teach the left brain and only the left brain learns. Teach the right brain and both brains learn."

Now, comes the tricky point. Visualizers are more often than not listening-learners. They simply cannot analyze well at early ages (until junior high, or so) because they have not yet developed that faculty. What they see, teamed with what they hear, constitutes their entire range of learning input stimuli. T h e s e stimuli are internalized holistically. Analytical processes are being developed all along, but slowly and with difficulty.

One point MUST AGAIN BE MADE CLEAR about teaching persons HOW TO THINK. IT MUST be remembered that this is something we CANNOT DO. People already know how to think from birth. They are already predominantly analyzers or visualizers with all shades of extremes and intermediate traits and combinations.

What we can do is to sharpen these innate faculties. That's where *art* comes in as an aid to visualizing and *mathematics* an aid to analyzing, for example. And the teaching of science HAS IT ALL: counting, measuring, data gathering and processing, infering and predicting—only to mention a few of the tools of thought.

Indeed, even those individuals blessed with extreme abilities for analyzing may be able to use these left-brain faculties for visualizing. However, there is more evidence that visualizing individuals can use their right-brain faculties to read and to do mathematical operations (analyzing).

It is likely that extremely left-brained individuals can probably teach themselves how to be better visualizers (that would be the only way that they would achieve these skills —by teaching themselves). However, there is less emperical evidence for this than there is for extremely right-brained individuals (listening-learners) overcoming these difficulties by junior high school age and thereafter being "normal" students.

Even in the best of special education programs, a large number of these children have been neglected for so long that "catching up" becomes a major obstacle.

For academic consideration only, it should be obvious that children with extremely strong analyzing abilities also could have problems. They too could end up in learning disability classes. While these individuals are probably few and far between, this statement is made to encompass all probabilities and invite further investigation.

Teach the left brain and only the left brain learns. Teach the right brain and both brains learn. Teach children to analyze and analyzing is all you've achieved. Teach children to visualize and you've also taught them to visualize and analyze. Teaching in the affective domain seems to do the latter.

From all that research tells us about how humans learn, this is certainly applicable in the education of children. It is less certain if this principle also applies to the education of adults. Cursory evidence is that it applies at all levels of human education.

SKILLS AND PRINCIPLES

1. The end product of human hemisphericity is that some individuals are innately analyzers and others are innately visualizers.

81

2. Teachers cannot teach children HOW TO THINK. They already know how to do that in their own way.
3. Individuals with two left hemispheres can teach or train these hemispheres to do right-brain functions.
4. Individuals with two right-brain hemispheres can train these hemispheres to do left brain functions.

Chapter 19

Listening-Learners
The Visualizer's Tool

While all students in any given classroom could be classified as average or active listeners as they learn, visualizing students MUST make an extra effort to be sensitive listeners. Coupled with seeing, listening is all that they have. During the formative years, what is simultaneously shown and talked about will be their most effective modes of input of educational data.

During the early years as a learner, the visualizer may acquire an acute and sensitive "listening-learner" mode of coping with his academic environment. Show-and-tell activities are great. However, as learners get older, the showing and the telling become separated.

Unless the visualizer's ears become as acute as his eyes, mental pictures and holistic vision may lag to create learning disabilities. Unfortunately, there are many other factors that contribute to the degree to which an individual may develop toward his potentials.

Given ideal conditions, the early years of reading education are highly visual. Visualizers can do quite well and can appear to be progressing right along with the analyzers. Analyzers prosper from show-and-tell lessons as well.

However, as the analyzers progress through what is as-

83

sumed to be normal development, reading develops without too much pain and strain. Not so for visualizers. They begin to stagger. Their listening habits are at stake. Success or failure, respectively, could either make the day for them or, worse, leave them with negative feelings about themselves.

Under ideal conditions, the sensitive teacher will see to it that the visualizer has opportunities to "talk" his way into some kind of success. Ideally, the visualizer will be made to feel that he is having difficulty with the activities—but not, however, as a result of inadequacies within himself. Nor should he be made to feel that he is less than normal for being slow at learning to read or doing other academic skills.

The vast number of students in all classrooms could learn to read quite well and effectively if they were all treated as though they were all visualizers (remember, "teach the left brain and only the left brain learns").

The only ones that would not prosper from this approach would be students on the two extremes—the acute analyzer because he probably already knows how to read (just a few of these—5 percent at the most) and the acute visualizer because he will not be able to cope with the symbolism of words for several years perhaps.

The acute visualizer will probably not do well because he is relatively incapable of grasping this level of symbolism at this point in his development. However, his right-brained listening abilities should be sensitive and acute. With patience and care on the part of the teacher, this should be his saving skill for these few trying years.

There is evidence that acute visualizers can be taught to read—even if they have to teach themselves. Perhaps this is where special education efforts could support these learners and their teachers through healthy and positive progress, as slow as it might be. With a good feeling about themselves, and as long as they remain relatively close to the peer group, by middle or junior high school age, they should be well prepared to cope with the best of analyzers.

Note that the emphasis is made on the individual retaining a positive attitude about learning and about himself and

84

remaining within and a part of his/her peer group. The condition of slow progress is usually temporary.

With less than ideal conditions, a human being can be made to feel like something less than a human. Worse, physical separation from the peer group becomes progressively wider as the individual progressively separates academically from the peer group.

Ability grouping may breed conditions where "good" and "bad" students—"bright" and "dull" individuals—are identified publicly. "This is the "A" group—this is the "Z" group . . . they can't learn . . . " Which, of course, is BAD PEDAGOGY.

Listening is the only tool that many learners have with which to defend themselves for the first few years of education. What more can we say than the condition is temporary? There are more justifications for "mainstreaming" of elementary school children than there are for "sidelining" them in any form of the so-called "ability grouping" commonly found in educational systems where the acquisition of knowledge is slanted in favor of left-hemispheric applications with little consideration for the affective domain.

When we consider visualizers as having acute listening abilities, this appears to justify "lecturing" as a mode of education. NOT SO. There are, of course, those excellent lecturers who one hundred percent of the time, or nearly so, seem to consistantly paint a "pretty picture" with words.

Such a person probably gets his point across to most of his students most of the time. However, these individuals are so rare that they should be considered exceptions to the rule. The rule probably is that each teacher has a "good" lecture, from time to time—some more times than others.

These exceptional lectures are those in which the teacher has a personal investment. Human interest stories are told to enhance the lesson being taught. Thus, a vivid oral communication is delivered, leaving all or most learners with a good and satisfying experience. The affective domain has served the individual toward a higher cognitive achievement.

Yet another academic situation presents itself with respect

to the plight of the listening-learner. Given an individual with a highly dominant sense of visualization, what would be the result of such an individual having impaired listening abilities due to defective ears?

Is one's listening ability made even more acute if his vision is impaired due to defective eyes? The same questions are asked about the results of an acute analyzer's personality development if he has an impaired vision or a hearing loss unchecked during the formative years. Definite and identifiable patterns would probably result.

Other considerations concerning brain lateralization and the relationships of visual and hearing acuteness would have to involve the role of the environment in the development of these traits. All talents have to be developed, or else they remain dormant.

The need for a close relationship between the classroom teacher and the special education teacher would seem rather obvious. However, when it comes to the development of a child's endowed traits, the third leg of the "important people" should also come into the picture—the parents. So, what else is new?

SKILLS AND PRINCIPLES

1. What are some activities that foster academic progress for both analyzers and visualizers?
2. What are some classroom activities that are good for analyzers, but could create difficulties for visualizers?
3. Is the inability to learn to read a permanent or temporary condition? How could you tell if it is permanent or temporary (since the possibility exists that it could be permanent)?
4. Describe the learning environment in which listening-learners have an equal opportunity to gain academic excellence with analyzing learners.

Chapter 20

Humanistic Education: A System of Coercion and Motivation

There is yet another movement in education which has found its way into the hearts of some educators and the jargon of all. That is *humanistic education*. It take its name from the Middle Ages religions who were all things for all men.

The neohumanists are those advocating meeting the needs of all through a number of ways, systems and programs. As with most of the other contemporary movements, humanistic education means different things to different people.

As with these other different movements, humanistic education can be placed in the context of its basic action-and-reaction systems emerging from brain lateralization. Whether one is an analyzer or a visualizer will determine his views on humanistic education.

Probably the best way to approach this explanation is through its description as a system of coercion and motivation. A teacher's behavior in the classroom will basically result from which brain hemisphere is dominant.

The constructive teacher, an analyzer and at home with reading, writing and classroom verbalization, will lean heavily on the grading system for interpersonal contacts with his students. Grades become reward for some and punishment for others. Thus, since education is firmly entrenched in this

87

system, grades are without a doubt the most important of all levels and facets of teacher-student interactions.

On the other hand, the creative teacher, a visualizer, goes beyond the grade book for a description of students. For him, these students are indeed human beings and to label one a failure, after all, is to reflect on himself as a teacher. He has himself failed to reach this individual failing student.

So that these extremes may be seen, with all shades of possibilities in between, humanistic education can be described in its dichotomy of behaviors based on the creative-construction model as well as on the two brain hemispheres (see Figure 7). It becomes a system of motivation for some and benevolent coercion for others.

Through the eyes of constructive individuals, or analyzers, humanistic education is deeply entrenched in the grading system. An A is, of course, the strongest means of motivation possible. An F is seen as a means of coercion.

If the teacher is hung up on the grade and cannot get beyond the grade book when discussing the scholastic progress of a student, there is little concern or understanding of "humanism in education." However, many of these teachers are indeed concerned with the human being standing at the other end of this stroke of the pen.

If grading is merely a matter of bookkeeping, everything is accurately recorded and transmitted without regard to intervening circumstances. Yet, grading *can* be done with care and compassion for the individual on the negative side of the grading spectrum.

This is perhaps why the two brain hemisphere, as prime movers of behavior, have eluded the scrutiny of analysis for the education system. There can be analyzers, steeped in the grading system, with feelings, care, and compassion for individuals. These teachers are, indeed, humanists in every sense of the word.

They scoff at the "bleeding hearts" of the movement who cry for the dismantling of the grading system. The analyzer teacher and the student are both aware that they have *failed*.

88

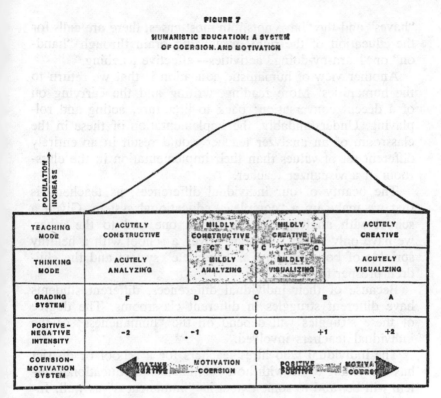

FIGURE 7

HUMANISTIC EDUCATION: A SYSTEM
OF COERSION AND MOTIVATION

TEACHING MODE	ACUTELY CONSTRUCTIVE	MILDLY CONSTRUCTIVE	MILDLY CREATIVE	ACUTELY CREATIVE
THINKING MODE	ACUTELY ANALYZING	MILDLY ANALYZING	MILDLY VISUALIZING	ACUTELY VISUALIZING
GRADING SYSTEM	F	D	C	B	A
POSITIVE - NEGATIVE INTENSITY	-2	-1	0	+1	+2
COERSION - MOTIVATION SYSTEM	NEGATIVE MOTIVATION / NEGATIVE COERSION		POSITIVE MOTIVATION / POSITIVE COERSION	

Viewed from a position that brain lateralization is a prime mover, humanistic education is a system of motivation and coercion. The dichotomous nature of these psychological structures are pressured by social, political, and religious structures—structures beyond the scope of these discussions.

And a bond of love and devotion can exist and be kindled by a caring and compassionate analyzer teacher.

On the other hand, most visualizer teachers have difficulties with the grading system. Grades are calculated from activities and examinations in much the same way as in the classroom of an analyzing teacher. The educational system demands this of such a teacher. However, there is a whole different system of values in operation.

In the literature, humanistic education ties in well with brain lateralization as it is concerned with the academic

89

"haves" and the "have nots." In most cases, there are calls for the education of the right, visualizing brain through "hand-on" or "learn-by-doing" activities—affective teaching.

Another view of humanistic education is that we return to the humanities. More reading, writing and the carrying on of a decent conversation: back to literature, acting and rol-playing. Understandably, the implementation of these in the classroom of an analyzer teacher would result in an entirely different set of values than their implementation in the class-room of a visualizer teacher.

The beauty of our individual differences, as teachers, is that we make up a "complete" educational system. Given a school with analyzer teachers from one end to the other, we have only "half" a system. Given a school with a healthy sprinkle of both, we have a "complete" system and the chil-dren prosper from it.

Because of their individual differences, different students have different struggles in different classrooms. The degree of these struggles will depend on the "humaneness" of the individual teachers involved.

The individual who hires teachers for a school or district has everything to do with how "complete" an educational sys-tem will be, and to some extent its "humaneness" as well. In-deed, this is too great a task to be left in the hands of one individual.

SKILLS AND PRINCIPLES

1. Identify the dichotomies of "humanistic" education.
2. Define humanism and neohumanism.
3. Relate the creative-constructive model with human hemisphericity.
4. Describe a "complete" or holistic schooling atmosphere.

Chapter 21

Quality vs. Quantity in Classroom Instruction

There exists a strongly polarized dichotomy of teaching strategies in the parameters of *quality* and *quantity* in classroom instruction. However, one must first get past jargon and semantics in order to uncover the delicate differences in practice and meaning.

A confusing factor is that one cannot exist without the other. Any teaching strategy will have a certain quality and can thus be quantified. Conversely, it can be quantified and will thus exhibit a subjective quality.

Thus, it is all a matter of degree, definition, and semantics. Some teaching modes rely more heavily on "quality-strategies," related with the affective domain, while others rely on "quantity-strategies,"related with cognitive achievement.

Quantity-strategies. By way of the most commonly practiced teaching mode (the so-called traditional mode) "quantity-strategies" means "materials taught are materials learned." The materials that are covered in class are seldom ever seen as anything less than having been thoroughly understood by the entire class "with the same quality of understanding" in all students.

Thus, the quantity factor, "the amount covered," is of prime importance. The quality factor, "the degree of student

91

involvement," is of lesser importance. A confusing facet is that ONE student could ask a question—ONE question. This could be interpreted as greater *group* involvement—without regard to *what* was being asked.

Individual differences in students are seldom considered. Indeed, ability grouping SHOULD HAVE (prior to this point in time) separated the "listeners from the non-listeners." Listeners are good students and the non-listeners are poor students. "Ability" grouping is a requirement for the ultimate success of this mode of education. Note that in this context the "good listener" is the analyzing student, at home with the 3 Rs.

Also, motivation activities may or may not be a vital part of this teaching strategy. Motivation could range from an introduction: "Today-we-will-talk-about," or a "right brain" experience like showing pictures and the teacher discussing them, or a teacher-performed demonstration.

Quantity-strategies, in the traditional context, result in a certain amount of materials having to be covered in a certain amount of time—there is always more to come in the next lesson.

These are the teacher's plans and they MUST BE covered at all cost. There is MUCH EMPHASIS on prerequisites. THIS lesson precedes THAT one.

Quantity-instruction always yields a subjective quality, to some degree. During the presentation, students may ask questions, make comments, or the teacher may ask leading questions through pertinent mental considerations. The level of student participation could be quite high. The quality-strategy, in this case, yields motivation, comprehension, and a healthy atmosphere of students satisfaction with these proceedings. Affective teaching has lead to a high degree of cognitive achievement.

It is under these circumstances that quantity and quality become confusing and difficult to establish as a dichotomy in education. However, the important questions to ask are: Is it a teacher-centered or student-centered lesson plan? If it

92

is teacher-centered and achieving a high level of quality, the quantity-strategy has also yielded a high level of success.

Ask, further: Were the discussions led by the teacher or by the students? Were all of the students free to participate? Were all of their comments accepted, incorporated, and used to lead the group to students' choices—or where the teacher wanted it to go?

Quality-strategies. It is clear that in the student-centered classroom, "how much" material to cover takes a back seat to topics that are important and of immediate concern to the students. Quality becomes a measure of "how many" of the students are so motivated as to be involved in the day-to-day educational process.

A quantity-strategy for the student-centered teacher could mean how many topics have been covered. However, this is a minor consideration and that strategy could be deemed *unfavorable*. The major consideration is "how many" students are actively involved in the process of learning. This kind of "quantity" in a strategy is favorable.

Quantity vs Quality. Recognizably, an eclectic teacher can pull in both of these extremes. Therefore, as with other para-meters, the academic importance of these discussions for the eclectic teacher is merely to render a better understanding of the extremes. This teacher may, from these discussions, come to the conclusion that one or the other of the qualities has been neglected.

When one asks the right questions, one begins to see a healthy blend of quantity and quality in one's own teaching strategies. Any teacher of any philosophy can have both—it takes some "bending" on the part of all, however, different bending for different teachers.

In this dichotomy, as with previous ones discussed, it is again pointed out that very few persons actually find comfort in either of the extreme positions. However, they (the extremes) do exist and so do the "tendencies" in some teachers.

In that regard, these considerations are vitally important to all teachers. Not that one is concerned about the extremes, but about one's own tendencies. However, it is through the understanding of these extremes that we will come to grips with the tendencies.

Hence, the differences lie in the subject-centered teacher seeing quantity as having to cover "X" number of topics (the cognitive domain). Quality is how deeply involved the students are (the affective domain). Note that quality is an added feature when students ask questions or in some other way show interest.

Notably, if one student asks a question, it is generally interpreted as having come from the entire group and that the entire group had the same concern. THIS IS criticism leveled by the student-centered teacher for this mode of education.

For the student-centered teacher, quantity means how many students are turned on to the topic at hand and quality means how deeply involved they are in the process of learning for themselves. THE CRITICISM from the teacher-centered teacher is that these students did not learn as many topics.

BOTH STRATEGIES work. With little bending, teachers on both sides of the dichotomy are better off bending a little toward the middle. By so doing, they fuse quality and quantity in a healthy blend for the maximum success of the students that are involved. Most teachers are eclectic and capable of implementing such a hybrid program.

SKILLS AND PRINCIPLES

1. Distinguish quantity and quality in instruction strategies as defined by
   a. An authoritarian teacher.
   b. A self-directed teacher.
   c. An eclectic teacher.
2. How can teachers of all philosophies best serve their students for the most productive results?

Chapter 22

Educating the Two Brain Hemispheres

Educating the Left Brain Hemisphere: Objectives in the Cognitive Domain. We already know how to educate the left brain hemisphere and do quite well in stimulating lingual, linear, logical and abstract mental data processing. This is done through reading, writing and arithmetic education.

However, there are pedagogical problems is so doing. We spend more time and effort teaching the three "Rs," as it is commonly expressed, than in doing any other efforts in education. Sometimes this seems to be a losing battle.

The problem lies in the fact (and there is no hesitation in calling it a fact) that there is the need to include the right hemisphere in this learning process. Indeed, evidence is that if we educate the left hemisphere, only the left hemisphere learns (cognitive achievement). However, if we educate the right hemisphere, both hemispheres learn (greater cognitive achievement through affective teaching).

Therefore, the question is HOW TO educate the right hemisphere as to gain this more complete learning experience. A little background of information is needed, first to convince EVERY TEACHER that there is indeed the need to educate the right brain at all!

Why educate the right Brain Hemisphere. Some persons

95

do very well in the "traditional" left-hemisphere input educational environment. This academic environment is healthy (so it is believed) for the "academically inclined" students.

It is proposed here that these so-called academically inclined individuals suffer, to some degree, in the traditional setting. Both brain hemispheres are in need of development. These students are in need of having their mental horizons expanded into "visual-spatial" capabilities, as well.

It is not sufficient that we "train," "practice," and provide "skill development" for these students who already have a fair potential in this kind of learning. After all, this is within the realm of their potential. They were possibly born with these capabilities.

However, THE REAL MESSAGE is that these students are robbed of yet another avenue of potential development —their visual-spatial potential. Educators have traditionally DEMANDED the education of "the whole child" or holistic education. It hardly ever happens.

The truth of the matter is, if current trends in our data findings are correct, the education of one's visual-spatial facilities means more complete data handling, permanent (or at least MORE permanent) learning, and positive attitudes toward learning further.

This means that individuals with dominant visual-spatial potentials would be able to grasp the content being taught more completely and effectively. It also means that individuals with a dominant linear-logical potential would have to stretch their horizons toward their visualizing capabilities.

Because one has a dominant visual-spatial potential does not mean that the linear-logical potential cannot be developed as well. So, too, those with dominant linear-logical potential can, and should, be in an academic setting which will foster their visual-spatial potential. This is what was meant by educating the whole child—or holistic education.

What good is it to be able to analyze the world and not to be able to visualize it? Proof of this comes with the ability to communicate our perceptions.

If one can really analyze natural phenomena, one should

be able to communicate his perceptions to others. However, the process of analysis, alone, is insufficient input to be able to share one's perceptions with others.

Conversely, if one is able to visualize natural phenomena, communicating them comes a little easier in that there are more common means of expression—art, poetry, prose, drama, and others. For the analyst, there are but prose and mathematics with which to communicate his perceptions and discoveries.

However, unless the analyst has "trained, practiced, or had skills developed in visualizing," chances are that his communications skills have likewise been underdeveloped. This leaves him with only mathematics with which to express or to communicate his perceptions and discoveries.

The need exists, therefore, to have greater right hemisphere input as the norm when educating human beings. A swing all the way to one hundred percent on the right hemisphere would be as much in error as to have one hundred percent emphasis on the education of the left hemisphere. Although, when we consider the evidence that "if we educate the right hemisphere, both hemispheres learn," the error probably would not be that great.

Educating the Right Hemisphere: *Objectives in the Affective Domain*. Skills development in the "art" of visualizing is of prime concern when educating the right brain hemisphere of human beings. Everyone is potentially capable of the development of this skill, to different degrees.

Just as everyone is capable of developing linear-logical skills, to different degrees, so is everyone capable of development of their visualizing skills. By so doing, one becomes a more "complete" thinker.

In the classroom environment, there is the added feature of developing communications skills along with visualizing skills. If the student is expected to share his perceptions with others through the many forms of communications, then these communications skills all evolve naturally and concurrently. Too, a personality is developed.

This is why it is so important to include visual expressions in the total education of human beings. Thus, "totalness" or "holistic education" is the plea of neohumanists and advocates of accountability as well.

Teaching students "how to visualize" is commonly done in the elementary schools by teachers who tell students, when teaching spelling, "close your eyes and see the word." It is done in art when students truly express their images onto paper or canvas.

The right hemisphere gains potential development when students organize written and oral reports, form their own words. And, when words do not communicate, they are encouraged to go to the board and "show" what they mean. "Draw a picture." "Show us what it looks like."

By the same token, when a teacher explains something once, he should never take the second opportunity to explain the same thing. Let a student do it. Take time to go to the board and illustrate or demonstrate the concept in some way.

Speak often of the "mind's eyes." Ask students to express, often, what it is that they see in their mind's eyes. In such a class, writing comes easily—so does reading, in preparation for the writing. Both of the brain hemispheres prosper, especially if lots of pictures, sketches and diagrams are encouraged.

Classroom Management. Read *Introduction* again. It should make more sense after having considered the philosophical, psychological and sociological bases for teaching in the affective domain. Also, it should make more sense when you consider the nature of the human brain hemispheres and its implication on how we learn.

Enjoy a warm relationship with all of your students. They are precious humans—worthy of your deepest affections.

SKILLS AND PRINCIPLES

1. We already know how to educate the left brain hemisphere through reading, writing and mathematics education.

2. Educating the right hemisphere requires more visual experiences.
3. Educating the two brain hemispheres simultaneously gives:
   a. Deeper understanding of the materials presented.
   b. Training in data input, processing, and output for a better educated person.

Chapter 23

Locus of Control: A Function of Environment or of Brain Lateralization?

A number of recent studies have been directed toward a better understanding of the degree to which individuals accept personal responsibility for what happens to them. Reportedly, some individuals feel that their skills, competence, intellect, and abilities are placed into action to control their destinies. These individuals have what is called *internal control*. Others feel that their destinies are a matter of luck, chance, or being dependent upon powerful other people. These individuals are referred to as having *external control*.

For internal people, events are defined as a consequence of their own actions and are therefore under their own, personal control. For the external person, events are defined as being unrelated to their own behavior and are therefore out of (or beyond) their own, personal control.

Some researchers have found that the locus of control (L-C) of children in the classroom is related to social behaviors, personality, ethnic group and social class differences, parent-child relationships, and learning performance. All of these factors, with the exception of the last one, fall under the influence of the environment. The last one could be influenced by environment and/or brain lateralization.

Since some researchers have found L-C to be a viable personality characteristic, strongly related with achievement, attitudes, and IQ, it is worth prospecting for the possibilities of it being a function of brain lateralization—or at least bring in any way related.

It was found that those who depend on internal L-C behaved in such a manner as to indicate that their own efforts, skills, and competencies were responsible for any reinforcement they received. On the contrary, those who depend on external L-C behaved in such a manner as to indicate that fate, chance, and powerful others determined the reinforcement that they received.

Under the hypothesis that *reinforcement acts to strengthen an expectancy that a particular behavior or event will be followed by that reinforcement in the future,* the operational statement emerged: Internal L-C is the perception that either positive or negative reinforcement is a consequence of one's own actions and is therefore under the influence of one's own control. And external L-C is the perception that either positive or negative reinforcement is unrelated to one's own behavior and thus beyond personal control (Joe, Nowicki).

The results of these research efforts on L-C show little difference between males and females in the elementary school that has not already been shown concerning their IQs. The academic achievement and social desirability of children with internal L-C invariably end up head-and-shoulders higher than that of children with external L-C. Studies also show that external L-C boys have heightened anxiety over internal L-C boys. This parameter is not significant in girls.

The IQ of elementary school students was usually found to be only a slightly better predictor of scholastic performance than was internality of L-C. The indications are that L-C tests give comparable results as do IQ tests.

It could be predicted that a visualizer, penalized throughout several years of elementary school for being incapable of thoroughly coping with the analyzing environment, would more than likely admit that most of his actions are externally

101

prompted and that a powerful other person (probably the teacher) has a relatively absolute control over his destiny.

It could also be predicted that children with internal L-C who are analyzers have met with a fair share of academic success, behave and believe they have a rather good control of their own destinies.

It is suggested that L-C is a function of past success or failure—little more than that. If the tables were turned and it were socially and academically desirable to be a visualizer, it is predicted that visualizers would have internal L-C and that analyzers would have external L-C, predominantly.

SKILLS AND PRINCIPLES

1. Define locus of control (L-C).
2. List the characteristics of individuals with internal control.
3. List the characteristics of individuals with external control.
4. How does reinforcement affect internal and external L-C?
5. Discuss the possibilities of L-C being a function of either environment or brain lateralization.

Chapter 24

Meeting the Needs
of All Students

Most significant in any teaching mode, in reaching individual difference needs, is that some individuals appear to have their thought processes dominated by the right hemisphere. These individuals, while rather intuitive in their rationale (if developed), have a penetrating insight in many ways.

Others, those who process their data predominantly through the left hemisphere, are both verbally and sequentially rational (likewise, if developed). These are the traits of academic success by today's teaching methods.

Meeting the Needs of Different Individuals. As it applies to both teaching and learning, our educational system is dominated by instruction through reading, listening, talking, and writing. Unfortunately, these are all left-brained activities. In our present system, the non-verbal (and often non-mathematical, as well) right-brained student is discriminated against by having to conform to these left-brained operations.

Because of this, *all students* are being denied an opportunity to develop the full capacity of both sides of their brains. If an equal attention were paid to the implementation of right-brained activities, all students would prosper. As it is, left-brained students are only half-way served and right-brained students are simply not well served at all.

There is the need to develop content, teaching methods, and materials that are suited for both the right and the left brain in an equal manner. This can be accomplished through a strategy that is aimed at stimulating both brain hemispheres—teaching in the affective domain.

When written words on the chalkboard are accompanied with representative pictures or illustrations, a thorough verbal explanation or description should be given at the same time. This combination stimulates both brain hemispheres in an equal manner. This can be accomplished through a strategy that is aimed at stimulating both brain hemispheres.

The traditional adage applies well here: "A student forgets what he hears, remembers what he sees, and learns what he does." This meets the learning needs of all students, analyzers and visualizers. The cognitive domain is satisfied through the affective domain.

The listening-learner is again brought to mind because of the nature of visualizing individuals. Show-and-tell programs during early childhood education meet the needs of all students because of the effectiveness that they have in teaching those students who CAN BEST LEARN THROUGH WHAT THEY SEE AND HEAR. While the condition is temporary, it is real and must be considered if all students in that classroom are to grow to their full potentials.

This mode of instruction has been used for many years by early elementary teachers in their "show and tell" program. It should now be expanded to fit the needs of all students at all levels. One is never too old or too sophisticated to be taught through the stimulation of both brain hemispheres.

Why Consider Hemisphericity in Education? One should teach under the assumption that we cannot teach people "how" to think. They already know how to do that. Indeed, that's the basic foundation of individual differences. Individual differences fade away when different needs of different individuals are met by a particular teaching strategy. However, they are magnified when the strategy meets the needs of one segment of learners while at the same time becoming a burden for another segment.

104

Hemisphericity and I.Q. Hemisphericity also plays a role in the determination of I.Q. scores—actually a test of left-brained operations. The I.Q. test is a poor test of creativity —a right-brained operation. Indications are that a person's I.Q. can be changed with prescribed changes in experience. The emphasis of education, then, should be on providing a more balanced array of experiences for all children rather than attempting to improve and measure left-brained potential.

Both Brains are Best Taught in a Student-Centered Curriculum Which is Project-Oriented. It is well established that students at all levels learn best when they are actively involved. Learning must also be internalized for maximum retention. This strategy should also include a student-centered curriculum.

The student should play an active role in the selection of "what" is to be learned. Too, it should be project-oriented. This means that students will also have some recourse in the selection of their own activities.

Students may be permitted to design their own problems. Designing involves intuitive, creative processes. By designing and then solving their own problems, students are engaged in activities requiring both hemispheres.

The teaching strategy suggested stimulates both brain hemispheres. It is student-centered and project-oriented so as to engulf the potentials of all students into individually conceived learning activities. Cognitive achievement is fostered by teaching in the affective domain.

It is designed to take into consideration the fundamental needs of all students at all levels. Whether the student is dominantly right-brained or left-brained should be of no concern to the teacher. Rather, it should be the aim and effort of the teacher to use all possible means to aid all students to develop to their full potential.

SKILLS AND PRINCIPLES

1. The educational systems are dominated by instruction through reading, listening, talking, and writing.

2. All students are being denied the opportunity to develop the full capacity of both sides of their brains.
3. The need lies to develop materials which will teach both brains simultaneously.
4. Students and teachers alike are encouraged to "show on chalkboard" what they try to verbally explain. Use more visual aids.
5. Explain the relationship between hemisphericity and I.Q. scores.

Chapter 25

Holistic Education
in Action:
One Way To Do It

The Characteristics of Holistic Education in Applied Education. There are probably as many ways of applying holistic education as there are individuals with the desire or inclination to do so. However, holistic education has its most natural and coherent status under the guidance of a teacher who is himself a visualizer.

Holistic education has several characteristics which are uniquely intended to totally involve the learner in both the teaching and the learning processes. Since the learner is to be involved in the teaching processes, this means that he will, by necessity, have some input in the selection of the course content. And that involvement should further evolve into his actively teaching other members of the class.

On the learning facet of the teaching-learning processes, the student should select his own project in the fulfillment of a small part of the total course outline. He should collect data and materials whereby he develops some expertise in the topic he selects, commensurate with his and the academic maturity of the class. This means that he should be prepared to share his contribution to the total course outline or content with the class.

107

The six steps or phrases of holistic education (teaching-learning) are as follows:

1. Group selection of topics leading toward the outline of the course content.
2. Distribution of individual projects that essentially (or as much as possible) cover the total course outline or content.
3. The data- or material-gathering whereby the individuals go to the four-winds and bring together the course.
4. The organization of the course outline specifying individuals' names, their topics, and dates of presentation (the course agenda).
5. Presentations by individuals as the specified course outline unfolds, day-by-day.
6. Student involvement in the examinations and/or evaluations of materials learned (formulating examinations and the application of these instruments toward grade assessment of the individual's progress).

1. *The Selection of Topic Outline for the Course Content.* Introduce the course in terms of desirable goals to be "covered," content to be learned, and procedures by which these goals and content are to be achieved. Set the pace for the students. Draw the content boundaries.

2. *Distribution of Individual Projects.* All of the students are to select a project that will in a small way lead toward the "coverage" of the total course outline or course content. They should know that they are selecting a topic for which they will prepare an oral presentation, with visual aids, for illustration, demonstration, or actively learning the materials of their topic. This is their responsibility to the group—as each of the others has what should be as much as possible an equal or comparable responsibility (or commensurate with individual abilities).

The method of delivery selected by students, in sharing these ideas with the class, should assist classmates to better understand and be able to use what they have learned in their

108

daily lives. This enlivens the affectiveness of the teaching strategy.

3. *Data- or Material-Gathering Phase.* Once the students know that part of the total outline for which they will be personally responsible, time will be needed to look up these ideas and to gather the materials necessary with which to illustrate, demonstrate or prepare class activities to deliver and share these ideas.

Send students out "to the four winds" to get these ideas and materials. The encyclopedia is just a starting place—not the only place. Review the introduction again, at this point. It will be helpful. These ideas will be invaluable in this MOST CRUCIAL PHASE of lesson-development.

4. *Organize the Course Outline Specifying Names, Topics, and Dates of Presentation.* Within a day or so of their involvement with their personal topics, have students start listing their names next to their topics so as to form groups of individuals with similar topics. Have the groups suggest dates that they will all (or most of them) be ready to present their topics to the class. As the course agenda starts to take form, make an attempt to start the first group as soon as possible, without rushing them to the point of sacrificing quality in their presentations. A "visible" copy of this agenda will need day-by-day adjustment.

5. *Individual Presentations.* As the day-by-day unfolding of the course agenda takes place, there should be a continuing atmosphere of "group satisfaction" as well as individual pride generated from these proceedings. Since this procedure will work with MOST groups, little needs to be said concerning pitfalls to watch.

However, groups differ and from time to time one will find an exceptionally well-disciplined group. On the other hand, there will be the occasional "inert" group that will take a bit more pushing and pulling (external and internal motivation). . . .

This should not take away from the quantity or the quality of the materials covered. Nor should it reflect the group or

109

individual achievement. Each individual is to be held accountable for his own achievement.

Discourage two individuals from doing exactly the same topic. It is too difficult to determine which person did MOST of the work. As long as each individual is accountable for a small, distinctly different, portion of the total outline, this will not be a problem.

Individual presentations can and should be assessed by the entire class. Organize a reporting system whereby the individuals can get "graded" by the group. Cut a stack of 8 x 11 inch paper into quartered leaflets (a good way to recycle used paper). Have students evaluate the presenters anonymously on these leaflets. By writing only the name of the presenter on each sheet, this assures that any strays will reach their destiny.

Each of the following criteria could be given a 1 to 5 rating ($1 = F$, $3 = C$, $5 = A$): 1) preparation, 2) oral presentation, 3) use of visual aids to assist in getting the ideas across, 4) how well the topic was covered, and 5) an overall grade for this person's project. Some groups will prefer a scale of 1 to 3 ($1 = F$, $2 = C$, $3 = A$). Another choice is to have a 3-criteria instrument: 1) preparation, 2) presentation, and 3) overall grade.

In all cases, when evaluating an individual, a very high mark (an A or a B) should be explained to show why it was such a good project. Likewise, a very low mark (an F or a D) should be explained to show why it was so deficient—it might even include tips on how to improve the next presentation.

The overall grade should be a reflection of the combined score for all of the selected criteria—an arithmetic mean (if the group is that sophisticated). Each presenter will then report these results to his teacher. In a two or three paragraph written statement, he would say: "Most of the class thought that my preparation was adequate. Their comments were . . ." "Several persons said that I should speak louder . . ." Don't overlook the character-building nature of these self-evaluations.

Ideally, as soon as the individuals have completed their

110

report to the class, they should begin their next project. Some students are at all phases of preparation at all times, having a few ready to present on any given day. However, this level of organization requires a rather mature group and should not be expected to work so well for each group. Best expectations are to lock-step the group through one unit at the time—all at the library at the same time, all presenting at the same time. The entire period, in this case, is devoted to whatever phase they are in.

6. *Student Involvement in Grade Assessment.* Some grades have been earned during the course of individual presentations. Assessing the achievement of individuals at the end of each unit of study is as much a part of learning as any of the other phases. Indeed, minor examinations in the interim should be learning experiences, as well.

It is possible for students to be involved with that aspect of their education, too. One way is for the announcement to be made that they will be participating with the testing process and to be prepared for a review. The review materials you gather can serve you well as the actual test questions. Or, at least, supply you with VERY GOOD ideas as you develop this evaluation instrument.

Have your students write three to five multiple choice questions, drawing the boundaries—from John's report to Mary's report. Or everything that was covered up to that point.

Write the stem of the multiple choice question and then PLACE THE CORRECT ANSWER IN THE FIRST RESPONSE, ADDING DETRACTORS as 2nd, 3rd or 4th detractors. Example: The sky is generally 1) blue 2) gray 3) red 3) covered with clouds 4) cloudless.

When reviewing, you have two volunteers (different two each time) to pick up the questions and read them thusly: "The sky is generally blue," read the next, and the next, etc. This will give them a very good idea as to what will be on the forthcoming examination. Make the test from these questions.

Sharing Visual Experiences. There is yet another practice which can be done at the end of any learning experience which will enhance the teaching-learning quality of holistic education practices. That is, upon completion of an important facet or phase of a unit, or the unit itself, have students meet in groups of three- or four-member discussion teams. The assignment: Discuss what you have just learned and draw a visual expression of it to share with the class.

Give ten to fifteen minutes for this activity. Early during the discussion, hand out colored crayons or felt pens and poster paper or sheets of newsprint paper. When time is up, have one person represent each group while another holds their visual expression, and discuss their collective impression of the learning experience.

While this cannot be done at the conclusion of all learning experiences, it certainly makes a nice change-of-pace activity while at the same time it holistically educates your students.

Accountability and Holistic Education. Students can set their own goals in course requirements, attaching grades to several levels of achievement—the essence of accountability. This way, however, the teacher guides the students into a hefty set of activities, upon the completion of which students receive As. With a lower set of accountable activities, those students earn Bs, etc.

The only precautionary measure recommended, or pitfall to watch, is that the list of activities should be challenging, yet realistic for the group at hand. Realize, of course, that groups differ and that the standards you maintain should bend with the group at hand.

See *Introduction* for further assistance in procedure and some suggestions concerning the content directions.

SKILLS AND PRINCIPLES

1. Organize your students into self-directed learning groups.
2. A self-directed class is a teaching-learning group experiencing holistic education.
3. A self-directed class is capable of maintaining group accountability in course achievement and grade distribution for various levels of activities.

112

Chapter 26

Facilitating Education

Education is a process which includes two acts: the act of teaching and the act of learning. The two acts need not be synchronized nor simultaneous activities. Many educators are yet to draw this conclusion and continue to have these expectations of their teaching activities.

Indeed, the acts of teaching and learning hardly ever have the types of connections listed above. However, because of different degrees of effectiveness and the efficiency of the teaching strategy, some acts of teaching more instantly, completely, and lastingly plant the seeds of learning in students.

WHAT is learned is not necessarily the content that was taught. For example, an arithmetic lesson (or geography, or any other) lesson may be taught. However, what was learned was to dislike arithmetic (or geography, etc.). For those unfortunate students, the next lesson may be even more difficult to learn and may reduce the product to a greater negativity.

Clearly, misunderstandings occur, creating misconceptions. Different individuals match the learned concept with personal past-experiencing, creating shades of different notions or visualizations of the learned concept. Thus, WHAT is taught HARDLY EVER IS what is intended to be taught for a number of assorted reasons.

The educator, if he wishes to be scientific about his teaching strategy, MUST account for this latitude in the learning

113

act. If his teaching act is to initiate effective and efficient learning, an accountable strategy MUST be devised to accomplish these objectives.

With shades of differences from teacher to teacher, the teaching act which MOST USUALLY reaps most effective and efficient results are those through which students learn more of the content taught while at the same time maintaining a healthy and positive attitude about the content learned. This accomplishment is A PRIME OBJECTIVE for FACILITATING EDUCATION.

"What topic(s) would you like to study?" "What would you like for others to study and share with you?" From these two questions, the course (or unit) content is developed. Students with similar interests are allowed to meet, plan, and to refine their own learning objectives. It is during this stage of development that the instructor has his last opportunity to make sure that the students' objectives (collectively) meet his own course objectives (objectives in the cognitive domain).

Motivating your Students. Be sure that they know that they will be held responsible to the group (class) for sharing their topic. Stress QUALITY in their teaching-sharing activities. When getting a point across, a picture is worth a thousand words (holistic education). Have plenty of newsprint paper and colored felt pens around with which to make diagrams, illustrations, graphs, sketches, etc. Help them to teach holistically.

There are yet other ways to achieve this quality of motivation in your students. One way is to announce the title of an upcoming unit. Then, pose the questions: "What do you already know about this topic?" "What would you like to know about this topic?"

Assign the task of writing an answer to both of these questions (about three to five minutes). Meet in groups of no more than six and discuss the composite results of their written comments for each of the questions. Have one person from each of the several groups to report to the rest of the class their composite comments.

You can make this activity more "group" oriented if you

114

write these comments on the board (in an abbreviated form). Add new ideas as they come up and place a check mark on the repeated ones—showing that they are so important as to have come up twice, three times, or more.

This teaching strategy is one that all facilitators will want to master. Again, the procedure includes: 1) Pose a pertinent or timely question. 2) Have students write or list their ideas concerning the concept, status, problem, alternate course, or solution to the problem. 3) Count the class off by groups of fours, fives, or sixes, so as to have no more than six in each group (a class of thirty members could be counted off by fives, giving you six groups with five members in each discussion group).

The amount of time to allow in these discussion groups will vary from topic to topic (and group to group)—depending on the nature of its timeliness in the views of the students. It can be observed that junior high school grouping and facilitating doesn't differ too greatly from that of college.

WHAT THEY ARE SAYING will give you the clue as to when to call time and end the discussion. At the first sign of their having exhausted the activity (they start discussing the upcoming football game, for example), give them another minute to complete their preparation so that one person may present their composite comments.

When you return their attention to the total group, there should still be the same interest in the topic that there was when they first broke off into their small groups. The fact that each group wants its ideas presented gives your topic new life—only to be exhausted, again, at the completion of the present activity when all of the subgroups have reported their comments.

The students will be anxious to hear what each of the other groups report. That is why you will want to keep track of each new idea as it is presented—and to check off the repeated ones. Now, take into consideration that this is the third time that each student has had an opportunity to adjust and readjust his thinking about the topic. This is QUALITY EDUCATION.

115

Some of the students may STILL want to make a bulletin board about the topic. Or they may wish to write a play about it (the seed being placed in responsible hands among your students). Maybe a newspaper article? Or TV and radio news? Exhaust all possibilities, leaving no stone unturned. Thus QUANTITY is enhanced with quality.

Facilitated education has several facets. Primarily, it is student-centered. No matter WHAT originated the learning act, or HOW, the student moves on his own motivation. He does something because he wants to. He is uncovering subject matter materials and information in his own way, his own time, and generated and maintained by needs within himself.

Another facet of facilitated education is that the learner has accepted the responsibility of sharing what he has learned with other learners. Each has learned different portions of a lesson plan, only to bring these portions together into a shared environment, one learner teaching the other learners. The lesser parts become greater wholes in different ways for different learners—each in accordance with his own experience-background input.

Facilitated education IS ALWAYS the act of learning which proceeds with self-motivated activities that end up being shared with others in what is often a culminating activity of that learning act. ANY teacher, with ANY philosophy, can achieve facilitated education. However, the frequency, duration and intensity of facilitated education will vary due to the philosophy and the value placed on the outcome, results, or end product.

Facilitated education does not take into consideration the cause or initiating act (the teaching act) that sets facilitated learning into motion. It is the quality of the learning act that identifies facilitated learning—self-motivated and student-centered. Therefore, it is important to consider HOW a teaching act can accomplish these objectives—these behaviors.

The classroom environment, obviously, must be an open atmosphere with a heavy flow of student input in the curriculum planning. It may originate with the teacher's plans.

116

However, they are shared with the students to the point that the students accept the plans as their own. The personal interests, background, and learning objectives of each individual fuse into a total consideration in these plans.

Class Attendance. Since the course suggested is to be humanistically oriented, a student who comes up with a valid reason for being absent and shows that he has read an article, should be allowed to share his reading with the class. Such behavior should gain for him full academic credit with the absence mark removed.

Impress the students with the fact that this range of behavior is not only tolerated but encouraged. Preach this and practice it.

There are untold social and psychological pressures on students at all levels of education. THEY WANT TO LEARN AND THEY REALLY DO WANT TO BE PROVIDED with a social norm in which they may function at ease and with the least amount of pressures and resistances.

However, the society does not allow for this smoothness in the lives of all—some are stressed beyond their own capacity to cope (even we teachers). Pray that your classroom is not one of those environments that place undue pressures on your students. This book has been dedicated toward making your teaching and their learning an intensely interesting thing to do. Students should be provided with a feeling of social ease in being with one another in your classroom. ONE NEITHER LOOKS (or speaks) UP TO OR DOWN TO ANOTHER. This is THE humanistic approach to education.

In a humanistic environment, the human person's attention and attendance in class is a matter of great importance. If the student is not attending your class, there MUST be a VALID reason. This is a "teacher's problem" that cannot be easily dismissed or handled categorically, and with a rigid set of rules.

However, there are some rules that can be proposed as a norm of behavior to which all students are expected to conform. One way to look at attendance is to reward perfect

117

attendance with an "A," to be averaged in with all other test and activities grades for the term.

A convenient and feasable way to do this is to allow each week of absence to lower the term grade by one letter. For example:

1) A class which meets each day, 5 times/week:

NAME	ATTENDANCE							
	A++	A+	A	A-	A--	B++	B+	B	B-
Student A	9/2	9/16	10/1	10/4	11/3	11/5	12/1	X
Student B	9/15	11/1	X					

2) A class which meets 3 times/week:

NAME	ATTENDANCE					
	A+	A	A-	B+	B	B-
Student A	9/2	10/1	11/3	12/1	X	
Student B	9/15	X				

3) A class which meets 2 times/week:

NAME	ATTENDANCE			
	A	A-	B	B-
Student A	9/2	11/3	X	
Student B	X			

NOTE: Student A receives a "B" in attendance in all cases while student B receives an "A." Student A missed the equivalent of one week of school this term.

The Textbook. A good way to look at the textbook is that "it is just about the only thing that all students have in common with one another." They all have a book.

Go to the textbook with the opinion that it is an excellent source of information. This information is readily available to the entire class. That makes the textbook a good diving board into the pool of all knowledge on any subject at hand.

Assign the various chapters of the textbook to student committees to "go through it and share those topics with the class that the author(s) wanted us to learn."

Again, go to quality learning. Have the students teach humanistically and holistically. You may even want to set up a way for the students to evaluate the presentations. Suggestions for doing this have been made in the previous chapter.

118

SKILLS AND PRINCIPLES

1. List the standing or universal objectives found behind the activities of a facilitaing teacher.
2. List ways of keeping students motivated in the learning activities as a facilitating teacher.
3. Describe one humanistic way to approach "the problems" that come with student attendance.
4. Describe one humanistic way to view the use of textbooks in the facilitated course classroom.

Bibliography

I. HUMAN BRAIN HEMISPHERICITY

Bakan, P., "Hypnotizability, laterality of eye movements, and functional brain asymmetry," *Perceptual and Motor Skills*, 28:927-932; 1969.

Bakan, P., "Right Brain Is The Dreamer," *Psychology Today*, 10: 66-68; Nov., 1976.

Blake, W. E., "Right-Left Brain Functions," *The Journal of Geography*, 78: 246; Nov., 1979.

Blackstock, E. and Gray, C., "Left-Hemisphere Damage—One Cause of Autism?" *Psychology Today*, 12: 34; Oct., 1978.

Bogen, J. E., "Some Educational Implications of Hemisphere Specialization," *The Human Brain*, Prentice Hall, Inc., Englewood Cliffs, N. J., 132-152; 1977.

Brooks, R., "Hemispheric Differences In Memory: Implications For Education," *Clearing House*, 53: 248-249; Jan., 1980.

Brown, W. S., "Left Brain, Right Brain," *Harper's*, 250: 120; Dec., 1975.

Buchsbaum, M. S., "Tuning In On Hemispheric Dialogue," *Psychology Today*, 12: 100; Jan., 1979.

Carmon, A. and Nachshon, I., "Effect of Unilateral Brain Damage on Perception of Temporal Order," *Cortex*, 7: 410-418; 1971.

Deglin, V., "Our Split Brain," *UNESCO Courier*, 2: 10-19; Jan., 1976.

Efron, R., "The Effect of Handedness on the Perception of Simultaneity and Temporal Order," *Brain*, 86: 261-284; 1963.

Foster, S., "Hemisphere Dominance and the Art Process," *Art Education*, 30: 28-29; Feb., 1977.

Frazier K. (ed.), "Hooked Handedness And The Brain," *Science News*, 110: 247; Oct., 1976.

Gainer, R. S. .and Gainer, H., "Educating Both Halves of the Brain—Fact or Fancy?", *Art Education*, 30: 20-22; Sept., 1977.

Gardner, H., "Strange Loops of the Mind," *Psychology Today*, 13: 72-81; March, 1980.

Gardner, H., "What We Know (and don't know) About the Two Halves of the Brain," *Aesthetic Education*, 12: 113-119; Jan., 1978.

Gazzaniga, M. S., "The Split Brain of Man," *Progress in Psychobiology*, Hall, Inc., Englewood Cliffs, N. J.: 89-96; 1977.

121

Gazzaniga, M. S., "The Split Brain of Man," *Progress in Psychobiology,* readings from *Scientific American,* 367-374; Aug., 1967.
Goleman, D., "Split-Brain Psychology: Fad Of The Year," *Psychology Today,* 11: 89-90, 149, 151; Oct., 1977.
Gordon, H. W., "Hemispheric Asymmetry and Musical Performance," *Science,* 189: 68-69; July, 1975.
Harris, A. J., "Lateral Dominance and Reading Disability," *Journal of Learning Disability,* 12: 337-343; May, 1979.
Hart, L. A., "New Brain Concept of Learning," *Phi Delta Kappa,* 59: 393-396; Feb., 1978.
Horn, J., "The Right Hemisphere Has Something to Say After All," *Psychology Today,* 9: 121; Dec., 1975.
Hunter, M., "Right Brained Kids in Left Brained Schools," *Today's Education,* 65: 45-48; Nov., 1976.
Hunter, M., "Two Brains of Man," *Clearing House,* 51: 196; Jan., 1976.
Kimura, D., "Cerebral dominance and the perception of verbal stimuli," *Canadian Journal of Psychology,* 15: 166-171; 1961.
Kimura, D., "Left-right Differences in the Perception of Melodies," *Quarterly Journal of Experimental Psychology,* 16: 355-358; 1964.
Kinsbourne, M., "The Ontogeny of Cerebral Dominance," In D. Aaronson & R. Rieber (Eds.), *Developmental Psycholinguistics and Communicative Disorders,* New York Academy of Science, vol. 263, 1975.
Kinsbourne, M., "Why Is The Brain Biased?" *Psychology Today,* 12: 150; May, 1979.
Konicek, R. D., "Seeking Synergism for Man's Two Hemisphere Brain," *Phi Delta Kappan,* 57: 37-39; Sept., 1975.
Krashen, S. "Lateralization, Language Learning, and the Critical Period; Some New Evidence," *Language Learning,* 23: 63-74; 1973.
Krashen, S., "The Development of Cerebral Dominance and Language Learning; More new evidence," In D. Dato (ed.), *Developmental Psycholinguistics; Theory and applications,* Georgetown Univ. Press, 1975.
Krashen, S. D., "The Left Hemisphere," *The Human Brain,* Prentice Hall, Englewood Cliffs, N. J., 107-123; 1977.
Lackner, J. and Teuber, H., "Alterations in Auditory Fusion Thresholds After Cerebral Injury in Man," *Neuropsychologia,* 11: 409-415; 1973.
Lenneberg, E., *Biological Foundations of Language,* New York; Wiley, 1967.
McGarvey, M. T., "Right Brained Student," *Man/Society/Technology,* 37: 22-23, Dec., 1977.
Mebert, C. and Michel, G. (Herron, J., ed), *Neuropsychology of Left-Handedness,* Academy Press, 273-278; 1980.
Miller, J. P., "Educating the Other Side of the Brain," *Orbit,* 8: 20-22; 1977.
Molfese, D., "Cerebral Asymmetry in Infants, Children, and Adults; Auditory Evoked Responses to Speech and Music Stimuli," *Journal of the Accoustical Society of America,* 53: 363(A); 1973.
Nebes, R. D., "Man's So-Called Minor Hemisphere," *The Human Brain,* Prentice Hall, Englewood Cliffs, N. J.: 96-105; 1977.

122

Raina, M., "Education of the Left and Right," *International Review of Education*, 25: 7-19; 1979.

Regelski, T. A., "Music Education And The Human Brain," *The Education Digest*, 43: 229-230; Oct., 1977.

Rennels, M. R., "Cerebral Symmetry: An Urgent Concern for Education," *Phi Delta Kappan*, 57: 471-472; March, 1976.

Restak, R. M., "Brain Behavioral Differences," *The Education Digest*, 6-9; April, 1980.

Reynolds, C. R., Riegel, T., and Torrance, E. P., "A Bibliography for Interdisciplinary Research on Lateral Cerebral Specialization and Interhemispheric Integration and Processing of Information," *The Gifted Child Quarterly*, 21: 574-585; Winter, 1977.

Ryder, D., "Bringing Up Baby Again: Incomplete Dominance," *Times Educational Supplement*, 28; Jan., 1976.

Sackheim, H., and others, "People Are Really Two-Faced," *Time*, 12: 126, 129; Dec., 1978.

Saks, J. B., "Brain Research Offers Lesson in Learning," *Education Digest*, 45:2-5; April, 1980.

Sperry, R. W., "Cerebral Organization and Behavior," *Science*, 133: 1749-1751; June, 1961.

Sperry, R. W., "Hemisphere desconnection and unity in conscious awareness," *American Psychology*, 23: 723-733; 1968.

Sperry, R. W., "Left-Brain, Right-Brain," *Saturday Review*, 2: 30-33; Aug., 1975.

Thomsen, D., "Split Brain and Free Will," *Science Digest*, 105: 105-106; April, 1974.

Torrance. E. P., "Japanese Attitudes on Giftedness and Creativity," *Education Digest*, 45: 29-32; May, 1980.

Trotter, R. J., "The Other Hemisphere," *Science News*, 218-220; April, 1976.

Virshup, E., "Art and the Right Hemisphere-Art and the Left Hemisphere," *Art Education*, 29: 14-15; Nov., 1976.

Wheatley, G. H., "Right Hemisphere's Role in Problem Solving," *The Arithmetic Teacher*, 25: 36-39; Nov., 1977.

Wheatley, N., "Brain Hemisphere's Role In Problem Solving," *The Education Digest*, 43: 50-52; Jan., 1978.

Wittrock, M. C.,. et al. *The Human Brain*. Prentice Hall, Englewood Cliffs, N. J., 1977.

II. HOLISTIC EDUCATION:

(Open Education,
Humanism in Education,
Student-Centered Education,
Teaching Strategies in the Affective Domain):

Alexander, W. M., *Are You a Good Teacher?*, Rinehart and Co., New York, 1959.

Allen, D. W., *Controversies On Education*, W. B. Saunders Co., Philadelphia, London, Toronto, 1974.

Bagford, L. W., *Strategies in Education Explained*, Karlyn Publishing, Urbana, Ohio, 1977.

Bagley, W. C. and Marion E. M., *Standard Practices in Teaching* (The MacMillan Co., New York) 1973.

Bellanca, J. A., *Values and the Search for Self*, National Education Association, Washington, D. C., 1975.

Belth, M., *The Process of Thinking*, David McKay Co. Inc., New York, 1977.

Benderly, B. L., "The Multilingual Mind," *Psychology Today* 15: 9-12; March, 1981.

Bolton, N., *The Psychology of Thinking*, Harper and Row Publishers Inc., 1972.

Brown, G., *Human Teaching for Human Learning*: An Introduction to *Confluent Education*, Viking Press, New York, 1971.

Bullough, V. L., "Dissenting Thoughts on Intellectual and Creative Achievement," The Humanist, 40: 43-46; Jan./Feb., 1980.

Bush, R. N., *The Teacher-Pupil Relationship*, Prentice-Hall, Inc., New York, 1954.

Combs, A. W., "Humanism, Education, and the Future," *Education Digest*, 43: 17-19; April, 1978.

Davies, I. K., *Competency Based Learning*: Technology, Management, and *Design* (McGraw-Hill Book Co., New York) 1973.

Davitz, J. R. and Ball, S., *Psychology of the Educational Process*, McGraw-Hill Book Co., New York, 1970.

Doran, R. L., *Basic Measurement and Evaluation of Science Instruction*, National Science Teachers' Association, Washington, D. C.; 1980.

Eiss, A. F. and Harbeck, M. B., *Behavioral Objectives in the Affective Domain*, National Science Teachers Association, Washington, D. C.; 1969.

Frick, W. B., *Humanistic Psychology*: Interviews with Maslow, Murphy *and Rogers*, Charles E. Merrill Publishing Co., Columbus, Ohio, 1971.

Gowan, J. C. "Why some Gifted Children Become Creative," *Gifted Child Quarterly* 15: 13; Spring, 1971.

Greenleaf, W. T. and Griffin, G. A., *Schools for the 70's and Beyond*: A

Call to Action, National Education Association Center for the Study of Instruction, 1971.

Greer, M. and Rubenstein, B., *Will the Real Teacher Please Stand Up?* Goodyear Publishing Co., Inc., Pacific Palisades, California, 1972.

Guilford, J. P. "Creativity," *American Psychologist*, 5: 444-454; September, 1950.

Guilford, J. P. *The Nature of Intelligence* (McGraw-Hill, New York)

Harbeck, M. B., "Instructional Objectives in the Affective Domain," *Educational Technology*, 10: 49-52; Jan. 1970.

Hein, G. E., "Humanistic and Open Education: Comparison and Contrast," *Journal of Education*, 175: 27-37; Aug., 1975. 1967.

Hockett, John A. and E. W. Jacobsen. *Modern Practices in the Elementary School* (Ginn and Co., Boston) 1938.

Hyman, D. T., *Ways of Teaching*, J. B. Lippincott Company, New York, 1974.

Joe, V. C., "Review of the Internal-External Control Construct as a Personality Variable," *Psychological Reports*, 28: 619-640; April, 1971.

Lewis, G. M., *The Evaluation of Teaching*, National Education Assoc., Washington, D. C., 1966.

Lowry, R. J., *Dominance, Self-Esteem, Self-Actualization: Germinal Papers of A. H. Maslow*, Brooks/Cole Publishing Co., Monterey, California, 1973.

Lyons, C. M., "An Argument Against Administrative Classification Systems," *The Humanist Educator*, 18: 4-6; Sept., 1979.

Maples, M. F., "A Humanistic Educator: Basic Ingredients," *The Humanist Educator*, 17: 107-109; March, 1979.

Maslow, A. H., *The Psychology of Science: A Reconnaissance*, Henry Regnery Company, Chicago, 1969.

Maslow, A. H., *Motivation and Personality*, Harper and Row, Publishers, New York, 1970.

Meer, B. and Stein M. I., "Measures of Intelligence and Creativity," Journal of Psychology 39: 117-126; Jan., 1955.

Miller, B. S., *The Humanities Approach to the Modern Secondary School Curriculum*, Center for Applied Research in Education, Inc., New York, 1972.

McClosky, M. G., *Teaching Strategies and Classroom Realities*, Prentice-Hall, Inc., New Jersey, 1971.

Nowicki, S. and Strickland, B. R., "A Locus of Control Scale for Children," *Journal of Consulting and Clinical Psychology*, 40: 148-154; Feb., 1973.

Nowicki, S. and Walker, C., "Achievement in Relation to Locus of Control: Identification of a New Source of Variance," *The Journal of Genetic Psychology*, 123: 63-67; Sept., 1973.

Ogletree, E. J., "The Open Classroom—Does It Work," *Education Journal*, 93: 66-67; Sept.-Oct., 1972.

Pine, G. J. and Boy, A. V., "The Humanist as a Teacher," *The Humanist Educator*, 17: 146-152; June, 1979.

Pittenger, W. E. and Gooding, C. T., *Learning Theories in Education Practice*, John Wiley and Sons, Inc., New York, 1971.

Ripple, R. E., Ed., *Readings In Learning and Human Abilities*, Harper and Row, Publishers, New York, 1964.

Rogers, C. R., *Freedom To Learn*, Charles E. Merrill Publishing Co., Columbus, Ohio, 1969.

Rogers, C. R., *On Becoming a Person*, Houghton Mifflin and Co., Boston, Mass., 1961.

Sonnier, I. L., "A Model of Contemporary Philosophies Used in a Science Teacher Education Program," *Science Education*, 59: 221-227; April-June, 1975.

Sonnier, I. L., "Logic Patterns and Individual Differences," *Southern Journal of Educational Research*, 10: 136-150; Summer, 1976.

Sonnier, I. L. and Kemp, J. B., "Teach the Left Brain and Only the Left Brain Learns, Teach the Right Brain and Both Brains Learn," *Southern Journal of Educational Research*, 14: 63-70; Spring, 1980.

Swift, M. S. and Spivack, G., *Alternative Teaching Strategies: Helping Behaviorally Troubled Children Achieve*, Research Press, Champaign, Ill., 1975.

Thayer, L., Ed., *Affective Education: Strategies for Experimental Learning*, University Associates, La Jolla, Calif., 1976.

Torrance, E. P. *Explorations in Creative Thinking in Early School Years*. Bureau of Educational Research, University of Minnesota, 1959.

Weinberg, C., (ed.), *Humanistic Foundations of Education*. Prentice Hall Inc., Englewood Cliffs, New Jersey, 1972.